HASHIMOTO MADE EASY: COOKBOOK & BEYOND

Just 28 Days to Heal Your Thyroid, Boost Energy, and Lose Weight Naturally with Simple Recipes and Transformative Strategies - Perfect for Busy Lives

Mary Walker

COPYRIGHT

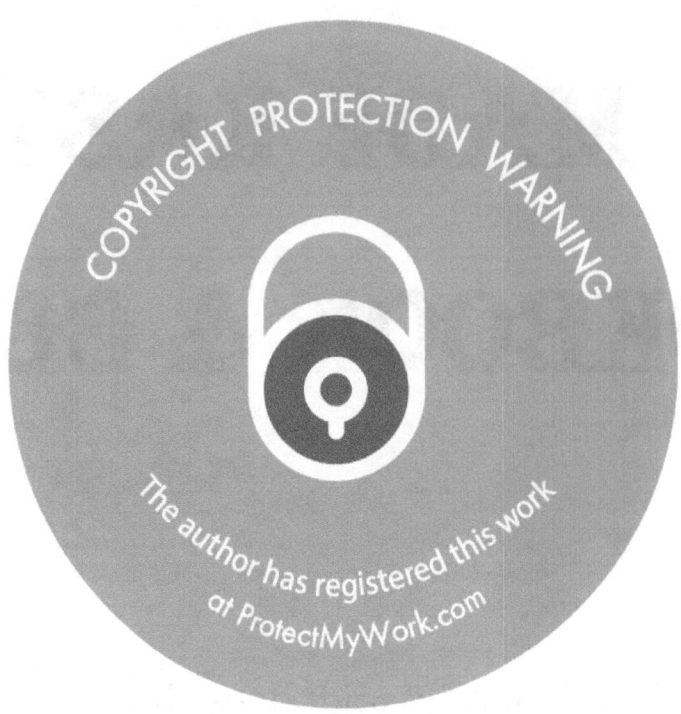

In no way is it legal to reproduce, duplicate, or transmit any part of this document electronically or in printed format. The recording of this publication is strictly prohibited. Any storage of this document is not allowed unless with written permission from the publisher.

All rights reserved.

The information provided herein is stated to be truthful and consistent. In terms of inattention or otherwise, any liability by any use or abuse of any policies, processes, or directions contained within is the solitary and utter responsibility of the recipient reader. Under no circumstances will any reparation, damages, or monetary loss due to the information herein, either directly or indirectly Disclaimer Notice: Please note the information contained within this document is for educational and entertainment purposes only. Every attempt has been made to provide accurate, up-to-date, reliable, and complete information. However, no warranties of any kind are expressed or implied.

The reader acknowledges that the author does not render legal, financial, medical, or professional advice. The content of this book has been derived from various sources.

Table of Contents

Welcome to Your Hashimoto's Guide ___1
How to Use This Book ___2

Part 1: Understanding Hashimoto's ___3
The Basics of Your Thyroid ___3
What Does Your Thyroid Do? ___4
How Is Hashimoto's Different? ___4
What Is an Autoimmune Disease? ___5
The Systemic Impact of Hashimoto's ___5
Recognizing the Signs ___6
Common Symptoms ___6
Common Misdiagnoses ___7
The Importance of Accurate Diagnosis ___8
The Root Causes ___13
Genetics, Environment, and Triggers ___13
The Role of Stress ___15
Nutritional Deficiencies ___16
Gut Health and Autoimmunity ___20
Hormonal Imbalances ___22

Part 2: Nutrition for Hashimoto's ___26
Food as Medicine ___26
Why Diet Matters in Autoimmune Conditions ___26
What to Eat ___27
Anti-Inflammatory Foods ___27
Proteins, Fats, and Carbs: Finding the Right Balance ___29
What to Avoid ___32
Gluten, Dairy, Soy: Myths vs. Reality ___32
Managing Sugar and Processed Foods ___33

Part 3: The Hashimoto's Cookbook ___35
Breakfasts ___35
Green Smoothie with Kale, Avocado, and Flaxseeds ___36

Tropical Smoothie with Pineapple, Ginger, and Coconut Milk _____37

Protein Smoothie with Almond Butter and Blueberries _____38

Almond Flour Pancakes with Natural Maple Syrup _____39

Coconut Flour Waffles with Fresh Berries _____40

Oatmeal Bowl with Chia Seeds and Cinnamon _____41

Spinach, Avocado, and Sun-Dried Tomato Frittata _____42

Scrambled Eggs with Mushrooms and Caramelized Onions _____43

Sweet Potato Toast with Hummus and Avocado _____44

Lunches and Dinners _____45

Red Lentil Curry Soup with Coconut Milk _____46

Seasonal Vegetable Minestrone with Bone Broth _____47

Baked Chicken and Vegetable Stew _____48

Slow-Cooked Beef Pot Roast with Root Vegetables _____49

Quinoa Bowl with Grilled Salmon and Lemon Asparagus _____50

Roasted Chicken Salad with Avocado and Sunflower Seeds _____51

Vegetarian Buddha Bowl with Spiced Chickpeas and Hummus _____52

Garlic Butter Shrimp with Zucchini Noodles _____53

Herb-Roasted Chicken with Sweet Potatoes _____54

Lemon-Baked Salmon with Broccoli and Cauliflower _____55

Beef Stir-Fry with Asian Vegetables and Ginger Sauce _____56

Spinach and Mushroom-Stuffed Chicken Breast _____57

Sweet Potato and Lentil Shepherd's Pie _____58

Eggplant and Chickpea Stew with Tomatoes and Spices _____59

Mushroom and Spinach Risotto (Dairy-Free) _____60

Lentil and Sweet Potato Patties _____61

Zucchini Lasagna with Turkey and Spinach _____62

Cauliflower Steak with Chimichurri Sauce _____63

Shrimp Scampi with Spaghetti Squash _____64

Salmon Patties with Dill Yogurt Sauce _____65

Thai Green Curry with Vegetables and Coconut Milk _____66

Moroccan Chickpea Tagine with Apricots and Almonds _____67

Indian-Spiced Lentil Dhal with Coconut Rice _____68

    Spanish-Style Garlic Shrimp (Gambas al Ajillo) _____ 69

Snacks and Sides _____ 70

    Energy Bites with Chia Seeds, Coconut, and Dates _____ 71

    Crispy Kale Chips with Olive Oil and Smoked Paprika _____ 72

    Homemade Protein Bars with No Refined Sugar _____ 73

    Beet and Tahini Hummus _____ 74

    Avocado Lime Dip _____ 75

    Spinach and Walnut Pesto (Dairy-Free) _____ 76

    Roasted Brussels Sprouts with Honey and Balsamic Vinegar _____ 77

    Grilled Zucchini with Garlic and Thyme _____ 78

    Mashed Cauliflower and Sweet Potatoes _____ 79

Desserts _____ 80

    Carrot Cake with Almond Flour and Coconut Frosting _____ 81

    Gluten-Free Brownies with Dark Chocolate and Avocado _____ 82

    Blueberry Muffins with Coconut Flour _____ 83

    Chia Seed Pudding with Almond Milk and Fresh Fruit _____ 84

    Banana and Almond Butter Ice Cream _____ 85

    No-Bake Cheesecake with a Date and Nut Crust _____ 86

    Baked Apple with Cinnamon and Chopped Nuts _____ 87

    Coconut Yogurt with Gluten-Free Granola and Honey _____ 88

    Dark Chocolate and Dried Fruit Bars _____ 89

Beverages _____ 90

    Ginger and Turmeric Tea with Lemon _____ 91

    Mint and Cucumber Infusion _____ 92

    Anti-Inflammatory Smoothie with Pineapple and Turmeric _____ 93

    Protein Smoothie with Spinach, Almond Butter, and Flaxseeds _____ 94

Part 4: Lifestyle Strategies for Thriving _____ 95

Stress and Hashimoto's _____ 95

    How Stress Affects Your Thyroid _____ 95

    Techniques for Stress Reduction _____ 96

Sleep and Recovery _____ 97

    The Role of Rest in Healing _____ 97

Exercise for Energy _____ 100
   The Right Workouts for Hashimoto's _____ 100

Detox Your Environment _____ 102
   Reducing Exposure to Toxins _____ 102

Part 5: Resources and Tools _____ 105
  28 Weekly Meal Plans | Shopping Lists _____ 105

  Conversion Chart: US Customary, Imperial, and Metric Systems _____ 111

  Conclusion _____ 112

Bonus _____ 113

Welcome to Your Hashimoto's Guide

First, let me begin by saying: **you are not alone.** If you're reading this, chances are you've been navigating the challenges of Hashimoto's thyroiditis—perhaps feeling overwhelmed, frustrated, or even unsure about what steps to take next. I'm here to tell you that it doesn't have to be that way. This book was created with one goal in mind: to empower you with practical tools, delicious recipes, and actionable strategies to help you regain control of your health and thrive despite Hashimoto's.

Hashimoto's is a journey, and while it may not be a path you chose, it's one you can navigate with confidence. This guide is here to simplify that journey, making it easier for you to incorporate meaningful changes that support your thyroid, reduce inflammation, and boost your overall well-being. Together, we'll explore new strategies, embrace small but impactful shifts, and create a roadmap for sustained health improvements.

What This Book Will Do for You

This isn't just another cookbook or health guide—it's a comprehensive resource designed to help you understand and manage Hashimoto's holistically. Together, we'll explore three core areas:

Nutrition: Learn how the right foods can become your allies in reducing inflammation, balancing hormones, and supporting your thyroid. From nutrient-packed meals to satisfying snacks and soothing beverages, you'll find recipes tailored to your needs. Whether it's an energizing breakfast to kickstart your day or a calming tea to end your evening, each recipe is crafted with intention and care.

Lifestyle: Discover how stress management, sleep, and exercise play a critical role in your healing journey. I'll share simple, practical strategies that fit into your life—not the other way around. These practices aren't just about addressing symptoms; they're about creating a life where you feel empowered and energized.

Health Management: Knowledge is power, and this book will equip you with the confidence to make informed decisions. You'll learn how to track your progress, recognize improvements, and celebrate milestones along the way.

Why Diet and Lifestyle Matter

Hashimoto's is more than a thyroid condition; it's a complex autoimmune disorder that requires a multi-faceted approach. While medication is often necessary, diet and lifestyle changes can significantly enhance your quality of life. Research shows that reducing inflammation, managing stress, and prioritizing nutrient-rich foods can help alleviate symptoms like fatigue, brain fog, and weight gain. By addressing the root causes and triggers, you're giving your body the best chance to heal and thrive.

Eating well and living intentionally isn't just about following a strict set of rules. They're about learning to listen to your body, understanding its needs, and making choices that support your unique health journey. This book provides the framework, but you hold the power to make it your own.

How to Use This Book

Navigating this book is simple and intuitive. Here's a quick guide to help you make the most of it:

Part 1: Understanding Hashimoto's – Get to know your thyroid, what happens when Hashimoto's strikes, and why a holistic approach is essential. This foundational knowledge will help you feel more informed and confident as you make decisions about your health.

Part 2: Nutrition for Hashimoto's – Dive into the science of food as medicine and learn about the nutrients your thyroid craves. This section also includes tips on meal prepping and selecting ingredients that best suit your needs.

Part 3: The Hashimoto's Cookbook – Find a variety of recipes for every meal, snack, and beverage, all crafted to be both delicious and supportive of your health. Each recipe is accompanied by practical tips to make cooking enjoyable and stress-free.

Part 4: Lifestyle Strategies for Thriving – Discover tips for managing stress, improving sleep, and building sustainable habits. You'll also find guidance on how to incorporate mindfulness and movement into your daily routine.

Part 5: Resources and Tools – This section simplifies meal preparation with detailed 28-day meal plans and shopping lists, guiding you to create balanced, thyroid-friendly meals. A conversion chart for US, imperial, and metric systems is also included for easy recipe adaptation.

Start Small, Think Big

Change can feel overwhelming, especially when you're managing a chronic condition. That's why I encourage you to take it one step at a time. Start with a single recipe, a new bedtime routine, or an extra serving of greens at dinner. Gradually, these small shifts will add up, creating a foundation of habits that support your health in the long run.

You don't need to do it all at once. This book is designed to grow with you, offering guidance and inspiration as you move forward. Remember: progress, not perfection, is the goal. Celebrate each step you take, no matter how small it may seem. Every positive choice is a victory for your health and well-being.

Take the time to explore each section of this book, and don't be afraid to revisit chapters as your journey evolves. Let this guide be your companion, your cheerleader, and your source of motivation. Let's embark on this journey together, one step—and one meal—at a time. Your path to better health starts here, and I'm honored to walk it with you.

Part 1: Understanding Hashimoto's

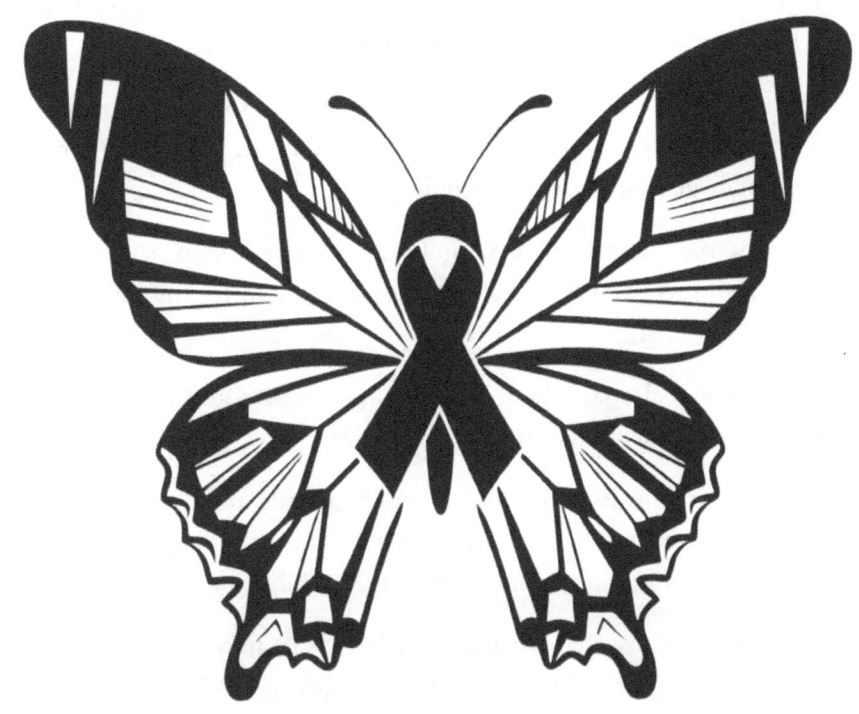

The Basics of Your Thyroid

The thyroid may be small, but it plays a big role in your body. Located at the base of your neck, this butterfly-shaped gland is like a command center for your metabolism. Its primary job? To produce hormones that regulate critical functions such as your body's energy levels, temperature, and how efficiently you burn calories. This unassuming gland is a powerhouse, quietly working behind the scenes to keep your body balanced and functioning optimally.

When the thyroid is working well, you probably don't think much about it. However, when its function is disrupted, as in the case of Hashimoto's thyroiditis, its effects can ripple through your entire system, impacting not just your health but also your overall quality of life. From subtle symptoms like low energy to more obvious signs like weight gain or brain fog, an underperforming thyroid can touch nearly every aspect of your daily experience.

What Does Your Thyroid Do?

Your thyroid produces two main hormones: **thyroxine (T4)** and **triiodothyronine (T3)**. These hormones affect nearly every cell in your body. Without these vital messengers, your body would struggle to maintain even its most basic functions. Here are some of the key processes they regulate:

Metabolism: Your thyroid controls the speed at which your body converts food into energy. This process directly influences your weight, energy levels, and overall vitality. A sluggish thyroid can mean a slower metabolism, making weight management more challenging.

Energy Production: The thyroid helps ensure your body has the energy it needs to function. When it's underactive, fatigue and sluggishness become a daily battle, leaving you feeling drained even after a full night's sleep.

Temperature Regulation: Ever feel cold when others don't? That could be your thyroid at work. It helps maintain your body's internal thermostat, ensuring you stay warm enough to function properly.

Heart and Brain Health: Thyroid hormones influence your heart rate and the efficiency of your cardiovascular system, ensuring your heart beats at a steady, healthy pace. They also play a crucial role in brain function, affecting everything from concentration and memory to mood stability.

In essence, your thyroid is a powerhouse that ensures your body's systems work in harmony. When something goes wrong with this gland, the effects can be far-reaching, impacting both your physical and mental health in profound ways.

How Is Hashimoto's Different?

Hashimoto's thyroiditis is not just a thyroid problem—it's an autoimmune condition. Unlike other thyroid issues such as hyperthyroidism or non-autoimmune hypothyroidism, Hashimoto's involves your immune system mistakenly attacking your thyroid tissue. Over time, this chronic attack can lead to inflammation and an underactive thyroid (hypothyroidism). It's this autoimmune aspect that makes Hashimoto's distinct and requires a more comprehensive approach to management.

Here's how it differs from other thyroid disorders:

Hyperthyroidism: This condition involves an overactive thyroid, leading to symptoms such as rapid heartbeat, anxiety, and weight loss. Hashimoto's, by contrast, typically causes the opposite: an underactive thyroid, resulting in slowed body functions.

Non-Autoimmune Hypothyroidism: This is hypothyroidism caused by factors like iodine deficiency or certain medications, but it doesn't involve the immune system's attack on the thyroid like Hashimoto's does. The underlying cause is different, which means the treatment and long-term management strategies also vary.

Thyroid Nodules or Cancer: These conditions involve growths in the thyroid and are unrelated to the immune response seen in Hashimoto's. While serious, they are distinct in both symptoms and underlying mechanisms.

What Is an Autoimmune Disease?

An autoimmune disease occurs when the body's immune system, which is designed to protect you from harmful invaders like bacteria and viruses, mistakenly targets your own tissues. In the case of Hashimoto's, the immune system sees your thyroid as a threat and launches an attack. Over time, this ongoing attack damages the thyroid, impairing its ability to produce hormones and disrupting its critical functions.

The root causes of autoimmune diseases are complex and can include a mix of genetics, environmental factors, and triggers such as stress, infections, or dietary sensitivities. While the exact cause of Hashimoto's may vary from person to person, the resulting impact on the thyroid is consistent: inflammation, reduced hormone production, and a cascade of symptoms that can affect the entire body.

Autoimmune conditions like Hashimoto's often come with additional challenges, such as increased susceptibility to other autoimmune disorders. Understanding this interconnected nature can be key to managing your health holistically and proactively.

The Systemic Impact of Hashimoto's

Hashimoto's doesn't just affect your thyroid—it impacts your entire body. When the thyroid is underactive, every system slows down, creating a domino effect of symptoms and complications. Common symptoms include:

Chronic Fatigue: One of the most debilitating aspects of Hashimoto's is relentless fatigue, making it hard to keep up with daily life. This isn't just feeling tired; it's an exhaustion that lingers despite rest.

Weight Gain: A slowed metabolism can lead to weight gain, even if your diet and exercise habits haven't changed. This can be particularly frustrating and emotionally challenging for many people.

Brain Fog: Many people with Hashimoto's experience difficulty concentrating, forgetfulness, and mental sluggishness. This cognitive impairment can affect work, relationships, and overall confidence.

Inflammation: Hashimoto's is inherently inflammatory, and this can manifest as joint pain, swelling, or a general feeling of discomfort. Inflammation also plays a role in many of the other symptoms associated with the condition.

Mood Changes: Depression, anxiety, and mood swings are common in Hashimoto's, as the thyroid hormones play a crucial role in regulating emotions and mental well-being.

The good news? While Hashimoto's is a chronic condition, **it is manageable**. With the right combination of medication, nutrition, and lifestyle changes, you can reduce the severity of symptoms and improve your quality of life. This book is here to help you do just that, starting with understanding the fundamentals of your thyroid. By empowering yourself with knowledge and actionable steps, you're taking the first step toward reclaiming your health and vitality.

Recognizing the Signs

Hashimoto's thyroiditis can often feel like an invisible condition, creeping in slowly with symptoms that are easy to dismiss or attribute to other causes. The subtle nature of its onset often makes it challenging to identify, especially in its early stages. Understanding these signs is a critical first step in taking control of your health and advocating for a proper diagnosis. When left undetected, the symptoms of Hashimoto's can escalate, making daily life increasingly difficult to manage.

Common Symptoms

While Hashimoto's affects everyone differently, there are hallmark symptoms that many people experience. These include:

Chronic Fatigue: A persistent sense of exhaustion, even after a full night's sleep. This fatigue can feel overwhelming and disproportionate to the activities of the day.

Sensitivity to Cold: Feeling unusually cold, even in warm environments. This can include cold hands and feet that never seem to warm up.

Dry Skin: Skin that feels rough, flaky, or unusually dry despite regular care. It may also be more prone to irritation or cracking.

Hair Loss: Thinning hair, brittle strands, or noticeable hair shedding. Eyebrow thinning, especially on the outer edges, is another telltale sign.

Brain Fog: Difficulty concentrating, forgetfulness, and a general sense of mental sluggishness. Tasks that once felt simple may become challenging and frustrating.

Weight Gain: Unexplained weight gain that isn't related to diet or exercise. This can feel particularly discouraging when efforts to lose weight yield little to no results.

Mood Changes: Depression, anxiety, or mood swings that seem disproportionate to life circumstances. Many individuals report feelings of irritability or sadness without an obvious cause.

Muscle Weakness and Joint Pain: Generalized muscle weakness and aches, along with stiffness or discomfort in the joints, are also common but less recognized symptoms.

Early vs. Advanced Symptoms

In its early stages, Hashimoto's symptoms may be subtle and easy to overlook. You might feel a little more tired than usual or notice your skin is slightly drier. These signs often blend into the background of everyday life and may go unnoticed for months or even years. However, as the condition progresses and the thyroid becomes increasingly impaired, these symptoms can intensify and multiply, impacting both physical and mental health:

Early Symptoms:

- Mild fatigue that feels manageable but persistent.
- Slight sensitivity to cold, especially in extremities.
- Subtle changes in mood or energy levels, are often attributed to stress or lifestyle factors.

Advanced Symptoms:

- Severe fatigue that disrupts daily life and feels insurmountable.
- Noticeable weight gain despite no changes in lifestyle or diet.
- Hair thinning or bald patches that affect self-esteem and confidence.
- Persistent brain fog and memory issues make focusing at work or school difficult.
- Increased sensitivity to cold that affects comfort and daily activities.
- Depression, anxiety, and a sense of emotional instability.

Recognizing these changes early and understanding the progression of symptoms can help you identify Hashimoto's and seek medical intervention before more severe complications arise.

Common Misdiagnoses

One of the challenges with Hashimoto's is that its symptoms often mimic those of other conditions. This overlap can lead to delays in diagnosis or even incorrect treatments, prolonging the journey to finding relief and effectively managing the condition. Here are some of the most common conditions mistaken for Hashimoto's and how they overlap:

Depression: Hashimoto's often presents with physical symptoms like cold sensitivity, dry skin, and hair loss, which are not typical of depression. Antidepressants may not address the root hormonal imbalance.

Fibromyalgia: Fibromyalgia is primarily characterized by widespread musculoskeletal pain, whereas Hashimoto's has more metabolic and hormonal symptoms identified through blood tests.

Chronic Fatigue Syndrome (CFS): CFS lacks the hormonal and metabolic markers of Hashimoto's, such as elevated TSH levels or thyroid antibodies, and does not involve physical symptoms like hair loss and cold sensitivity.

Perimenopause or Menopause: Menopause involves a decline in reproductive hormones, while Hashimoto's affects thyroid hormones and includes additional systemic symptoms like joint pain and weight gain.

Anxiety Disorders: Hashimoto's-induced anxiety is often accompanied by physical symptoms like weight gain, cold intolerance, and dry skin, which anxiety disorders typically do not include.

Vitamin Deficiencies: Deficiencies in vitamins like B12 or D can contribute to fatigue but do not cause the systemic hormonal and inflammatory changes seen in Hashimoto's.

The Importance of Accurate Diagnosis

Hashimoto's requires a specific diagnostic approach, including a detailed analysis of thyroid function through blood tests such as TSH, T3, T4, and thyroid antibodies (anti-TPO and anti-TG). These tests provide a comprehensive snapshot of how your thyroid is functioning and whether your immune system is actively contributing to the dysfunction. Neglecting these crucial tests can result in missed diagnoses, leading to treatments that only address symptoms—such as antidepressants for mood changes or painkillers for joint discomfort—while the root cause goes unaddressed. This can not only delay proper treatment but also exacerbate symptoms, making the journey to recovery more challenging.

TSH (Thyroid-Stimulating Hormone)

What It Measures: TSH is a hormone produced by the pituitary gland that signals the thyroid to produce T3 and T4 hormones. It serves as a feedback loop between the thyroid and pituitary gland, ensuring that hormone levels are maintained within a healthy range. When the thyroid is underactive, the pituitary increases TSH production to stimulate it.

How to Interpret It: Elevated TSH levels are a classic indicator of hypothyroidism, signaling that the pituitary is compensating for an underperforming thyroid. For instance, in Hashimoto's, elevated TSH often reflects the thyroid's struggle to meet the body's demands due to autoimmune damage. Conversely, low TSH levels may indicate hyperthyroidism, where the thyroid is overactive, or over-supplementation with thyroid hormone medication. Fluctuations in TSH can also be influenced by stress, medications, or transient thyroiditis.

What Persistently Elevated TSH Indicates: Consistently high TSH levels over time suggest chronic hypothyroidism, which can result in fatigue, weight gain, depression, and other systemic symptoms. It may also highlight untreated or inadequately treated Hashimoto's.

Normal Range: Generally, 0.5 - 4.5 mIU/L. However, many experts suggest that the optimal range for thyroid health lies between 1.0 and 2.0 mIU/L for those undergoing thyroid treatment. A TSH level above 4.5 mIU/L warrants further testing to identify underlying causes, while levels significantly above 10 mIU/L are usually treated with thyroid hormone replacement therapy.

Free T4 (Thyroxine)

What It Measures: T4 is the inactive precursor of T3, produced by the thyroid gland. It acts as a reservoir for the active hormone, meaning it provides a steady supply of T4 that the body can convert to T3 as needed. This process is vital for maintaining energy levels, regulating metabolism, and supporting other critical bodily functions. Without adequate T4, the body struggles to produce sufficient T3, leading to widespread symptoms of hypothyroidism.

How to Interpret It: Low T4 levels often indicate primary hypothyroidism due to insufficient hormone production by the thyroid gland itself. This is commonly seen in Hashimoto's as the autoimmune attack gradually reduces the thyroid's ability to function. Conversely, elevated T4 levels might suggest hyperthyroidism, which could result from conditions like Graves' disease, or over-supplementation with synthetic thyroid hormone (levothyroxine). It's crucial to analyze T4 alongside TSH to get a complete picture of thyroid function, as T4 alone cannot determine whether the thyroid is underactive or overactive.

Factors Influencing T4 Levels: T4 levels can also be affected by external factors such as pregnancy, stress, and certain medications, including corticosteroids and birth control pills. These factors can alter hormone production or affect how T4 is processed in the body.

Normal Range: 0.8 - 1.8 ng/dL. However, the interpretation of T4 levels should always consider individual symptoms and overall health. For instance, a T4 level on the lower end of the range might still cause symptoms in some individuals, requiring a more tailored approach to treatment.

Free T3 (Triiodothyronine)

What It Measures: T3 is the active thyroid hormone that influences nearly every cell in the body. It is converted from T4 in peripheral tissues, such as the liver, kidneys, and muscles. Unlike T4, which is a storage hormone, T3 is immediately active and directly impacts metabolism, energy production, and body temperature regulation. Its role is crucial for cognitive function, muscle strength, and overall vitality.

How to Interpret It: Low T3 levels may signal impaired conversion of T4 to T3, a common issue in Hashimoto's patients. This impaired conversion can occur due to stress, inflammation, nutritional deficiencies (such as selenium or zinc), or underlying chronic conditions. Even when TSH and T4 levels appear normal, low T3 can leave patients with unresolved symptoms like fatigue, brain fog, hair loss, or depression. In such cases, addressing the underlying causes of poor conversion, such as improving gut health or managing stress, can significantly enhance T3 levels and overall well-being.

What High T3 Levels May Indicate: Elevated T3 levels are less common in Hashimoto's but can occur in cases of overactive thyroid states or excessive thyroid medication. This condition, known as T3 toxicosis, may result in symptoms such as palpitations, anxiety, or unexplained weight loss.

Normal Range: 2.3 - 4.1 pg/mL. Suboptimal T3 levels might require lifestyle changes, such as adopting a nutrient-rich, anti-inflammatory diet, supplementation with selenium or iodine (if appropriate), or a combination therapy approach involving both T4 and T3 hormone replacements. Regular monitoring and follow-up are essential to ensure therapy adjustments meet individual needs and resolve symptoms effectively.

Anti-TPO Antibodies (Thyroid Peroxidase Antibodies)

What It Measures: Anti-TPO antibodies reflect the immune system's attack on thyroid peroxidase, an enzyme essential for producing thyroid hormones. This enzyme is critical for the synthesis of T4 and T3 hormones, as it facilitates the binding of iodine to the amino acid tyrosine, a crucial step in thyroid hormone production. The presence of anti-TPO antibodies indicates that the body's immune system mistakenly targets this enzyme, leading to chronic inflammation and progressive thyroid damage.

How to Interpret It: Elevated anti-TPO levels confirm the autoimmune nature of Hashimoto's, as these antibodies are a hallmark of the condition. These antibodies often appear early in the disease process, even before significant abnormalities in TSH or T4 levels. High levels of anti-TPO antibodies suggest active thyroid inflammation and ongoing autoimmune activity. It's important to note that the degree of elevation does not always correlate directly with symptom severity, but persistently high levels can indicate a higher risk of thyroid dysfunction over time.

Clinical Implications: The detection of anti-TPO antibodies can aid in distinguishing Hashimoto's from other thyroid disorders. For example, patients with elevated TSH but normal anti-TPO levels might be dealing with non-autoimmune hypothyroidism. Monitoring these antibodies over time can also help assess the effectiveness of dietary and lifestyle interventions aimed at reducing autoimmune activity.

Normal Range: Less than 34 IU/mL. Levels significantly above this threshold indicate active autoimmune thyroiditis. Extremely high levels, such as those exceeding 1,000 IU/mL, are often associated with advanced stages of thyroid destruction and may warrant more aggressive monitoring and management.

Anti-TG Antibodies (Thyroglobulin Antibodies)

What It Measures: Anti-TG antibodies target thyroglobulin, a protein crucial for thyroid hormone synthesis. Thyroglobulin serves as a building block for the production of T3 and T4 hormones, making it a key player in maintaining thyroid function. The presence of anti-TG antibodies indicates that the immune system is mistakenly targeting this essential protein, which can disrupt hormone production and lead to thyroid dysfunction over time.

How to Interpret It: Elevated anti-TG levels often accompany anti-TPO antibodies in Hashimoto's patients. While they are less specific than anti-TPO antibodies, their presence provides additional confirmation of an autoimmune process targeting the thyroid gland. High levels may indicate active thyroid inflammation and a heightened autoimmune response. In some cases, anti-TG antibodies may be the sole marker of an autoimmune condition, particularly in the early stages of Hashimoto's.

Clinical Implications: Elevated anti-TG antibodies can signal progressive thyroid damage, even if other thyroid hormone levels appear normal. They are also valuable in monitoring the progression of Hashimoto's and assessing the effectiveness of interventions aimed at reducing autoimmune activity. Additionally, persistent elevation of anti-TG antibodies has been linked to an increased risk of thyroid cancer in some studies, highlighting the importance of regular monitoring.

Normal Range: Less than 30 IU/mL. Elevated levels should be assessed alongside TPO antibodies for a comprehensive picture of thyroid health. When both anti-TG and anti-TPO antibodies are elevated, it strongly suggests Hashimoto's thyroiditis and warrants a comprehensive treatment plan focused on reducing inflammation and supporting thyroid function.

Why Comprehensive Testing Matters

An accurate diagnosis goes beyond symptom management. It ensures that the underlying autoimmune dysfunction is identified and addressed. For example, treating mood swings with antidepressants or joint pain with NSAIDs provides temporary relief but ignores the thyroid's critical role in these symptoms. Without proper diagnosis, patients often endure years of unnecessary treatments, increasing frustration and health complications.

Advocating for a full thyroid panel, including TSH, Free T4, Free T3, and both thyroid antibody tests, is essential. Many healthcare providers may initially overlook the autoimmune component, focusing solely on TSH. If your concerns aren't being fully addressed, consider seeking a second opinion or consulting with a specialist experienced in autoimmune thyroid conditions.

Understanding and Acting on Your Results

High TSH with Low T4/T3: This combination typically indicates primary hypothyroidism and often correlates with Hashimoto's. Primary hypothyroidism occurs when the thyroid gland itself fails to produce adequate hormones, often due to autoimmune damage. Hashimoto's-related hypothyroidism frequently presents this pattern, and it highlights the need for thyroid hormone replacement therapy. Treatment usually involves levothyroxine, a synthetic form of T4, which helps normalize TSH levels and alleviate symptoms such as fatigue, weight gain, and brain fog. Close monitoring is essential to ensure the dosage is effective and does not lead to over-treatment, which can cause symptoms of hyperthyroidism.

Normal TSH with Low T3: Poor conversion of T4 to T3 is a hallmark of non-thyroidal illness syndrome (NTIS) or under-conversion in Hashimoto's. This condition arises when the body struggles to convert inactive T4 into the active T3 hormone, which is crucial for energy production and metabolic function. Factors such as chronic stress, inflammation, or nutrient deficiencies (e.g., selenium, zinc) often contribute to this impaired conversion. Addressing this issue requires a holistic approach, including dietary support with nutrient-rich, anti-inflammatory foods, stress management techniques like mindfulness or yoga, and potentially the use of combination hormone therapy (e.g., adding liothyronine/T3 to levothyroxine).

Elevated Anti-TPO/Anti-TG: These markers confirm Hashimoto's, even if TSH and T4 levels are within range. The presence of these antibodies signifies that the immune system is actively attacking thyroid tissue, leading to inflammation and gradual destruction of the gland. Early detection of elevated antibodies allows for the implementation of preventive strategies, such as dietary changes (e.g., adopting a gluten-free diet), lifestyle adjustments, and stress reduction to slow the autoimmune process. Regular monitoring of antibody levels can also provide insights into the effectiveness of interventions aimed at reducing inflammation and supporting thyroid health. In some cases, persistently high antibody levels may warrant more aggressive management to prevent further thyroid damage.

How These Tests Fit into a Broader Wellness Plan

Recognizing the signs of thyroid dysfunction is just the beginning. Accurate diagnostic testing allows you to take proactive steps to protect and improve your health. Dietary modifications, such as adopting a gluten-free, anti-inflammatory diet, can complement medical treatment by reducing systemic inflammation and supporting thyroid function. Stress reduction techniques, adequate sleep, and targeted supplementation also play critical roles in optimizing thyroid health.

By recognizing the complexity of Hashimoto's and its potential overlap with other conditions, you're already taking an essential step toward better health. This knowledge empowers you to work collaboratively with your healthcare provider, ensuring that your treatment plan is tailored to your unique needs and evolves as your condition changes. Regular follow-ups and adjustments based on test results will help maintain balance and long-term vitality.

Next Steps for Your Health

Taking control of your thyroid health starts with education and advocacy. Armed with a detailed understanding of these diagnostic tests, you can confidently navigate conversations with your healthcare team. Combine these insights with dietary changes, stress management, and lifestyle adjustments to create a comprehensive plan for reclaiming your energy, optimizing your thyroid health, and achieving overall wellness. Your journey to vitality begins here.

The Root Causes

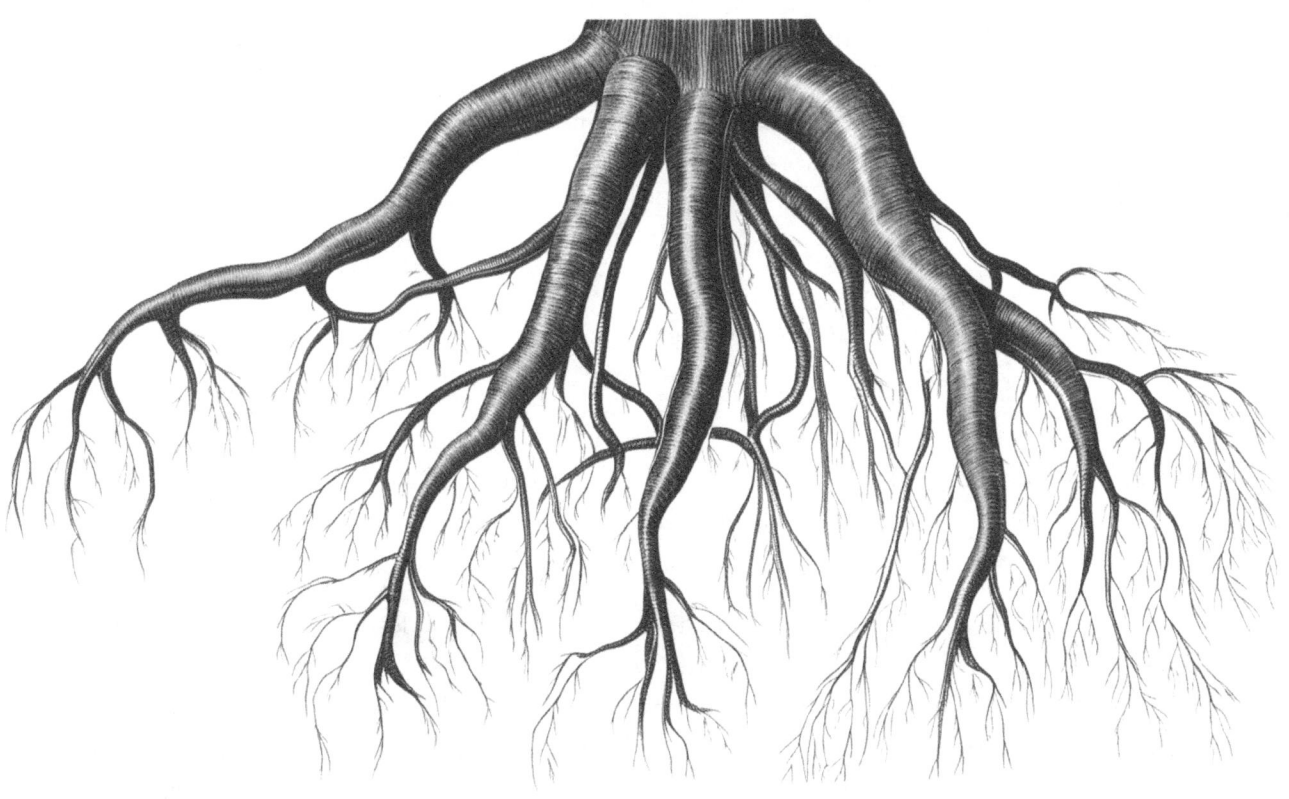

Genetics, Environment, and Triggers

Hashimoto's thyroiditis does not arise in isolation. It is the result of a complex interplay between genetic predisposition, environmental factors, and specific triggers that ignite the autoimmune process. These elements are deeply interconnected, with one often amplifying the effects of another. For example, a genetic predisposition might make an individual more vulnerable to environmental toxins or infections, while chronic stress can exacerbate dietary sensitivities or hormonal imbalances. Understanding how these factors overlap and influence each other can provide a more comprehensive view of the condition and highlight the importance of a holistic approach to management. Understanding these contributing elements can empower you to manage your condition more effectively and possibly mitigate its progression. A deeper awareness of these factors not only offers clarity but also highlights actionable steps you can take to minimize their impact.

Genetic Predisposition

Research shows that Hashimoto's often runs in families. Studies estimate that individuals with a first-degree relative affected by Hashimoto's or another autoimmune disease, such as rheumatoid arthritis or lupus, have up to a fivefold increased risk of developing the condition. Genetic susceptibility means you may be predisposed, but it is not a guarantee that you will develop the disease. Environmental and lifestyle factors often play the deciding role in whether the disease manifests, emphasizing the importance of proactive measures, even in the absence of symptoms. This connection underscores the importance of proactive measures, even if you have not yet experienced symptoms.

Environmental Factors

While genetics lay the groundwork, environmental triggers can push the immune system into overdrive. Common contributors include infections, toxins, dietary triggers, and iodine levels, each playing a unique role in the progression of Hashimoto's.

Viral or bacterial infections, such as Epstein-Barr virus (EBV) or Helicobacter pylori, have been linked to the onset of Hashimoto's. These infections can stimulate the immune system, sometimes leading it to mistakenly target the thyroid. Understanding and addressing past infections can provide insight into potential triggers.

Exposure to environmental toxins, such as heavy metals (e.g., mercury or lead), pesticides, and industrial pollutants, can disrupt thyroid function and contribute to autoimmune activity. These toxins can interfere with the delicate balance of thyroid hormone production by damaging thyroid cells and altering the gland's ability to absorb iodine effectively. Additionally, they may provoke chronic inflammation and oxidative stress, further straining the immune system and increasing its likelihood of mistakenly targeting the thyroid gland. These substances may accumulate in the body over time, gradually increasing the burden on the thyroid gland and immune system.

Certain foods can act as triggers for those predisposed to Hashimoto's. Gluten, found in wheat, barley, and rye, can exacerbate inflammation and intestinal permeability (leaky gut) in some individuals. Dairy products, particularly casein, can provoke immune responses in sensitive individuals. Refined sugar, known to promote inflammation, can worsen autoimmune symptoms and increase overall systemic stress.

Both excessive and insufficient iodine intake can impact thyroid health. While iodine is essential for thyroid hormone production, an imbalance can stress the gland and exacerbate autoimmune activity. Careful monitoring of iodine levels is critical, especially in areas where iodine supplementation is common.

Understanding Your Triggers

Identifying your specific triggers can take time and often requires a process of elimination. Working with a healthcare professional, such as a functional medicine practitioner, can help you pinpoint environmental or dietary factors contributing to your symptoms. Tracking symptoms alongside changes in your environment, diet, or stress levels can provide valuable insights, enabling you to make more informed decisions about your health.

The Role of Stress

Chronic stress is one of the most overlooked but impactful factors in the development and progression of Hashimoto's. While short-term stress is a natural and sometimes beneficial response, chronic stress can wreak havoc on your immune system, thyroid function, and overall health. By understanding the mechanisms through which stress affects the body, you can take meaningful steps to counteract its effects and protect your thyroid.

How Stress Affects the Immune System

When you experience stress, your body releases cortisol, a hormone that helps you respond to immediate challenges. This "fight-or-flight" response is designed to be short-lived. However, prolonged stress keeps cortisol levels elevated, which can suppress immune regulation, making it harder for the body to differentiate between harmful invaders and its own tissues. This confusion can amplify autoimmune activity, increasing inflammation—a key driver of Hashimoto's. Additionally, elevated cortisol levels disrupt the balance of other hormones, including those produced by the thyroid, further exacerbating the condition.

Over time, this chronic immune activation can worsen Hashimoto's symptoms and accelerate thyroid damage, creating a cycle that can feel difficult to break. Awareness of this cycle is the first step toward mitigating its impact.

Stress and Hashimoto's Symptoms

Stress doesn't just influence the underlying mechanisms of Hashimoto's; it can also exacerbate its symptoms. Chronic stress disrupts the hormonal balance needed for proper thyroid function by keeping cortisol levels elevated for extended periods. This prolonged elevation interferes with the thyroid's ability to produce and regulate hormones effectively, contributing to fatigue, brain fog, and other hallmark symptoms. Additionally, stress can weaken the immune system's ability to differentiate between harmful invaders and healthy tissues, amplifying autoimmune activity and inflammation. Many individuals report that periods of high stress coincide with increased fatigue, worsening brain fog, heightened sensitivity to cold, and more pronounced mood swings and anxiety. These symptoms can become self-reinforcing, as stress over managing symptoms often adds to the overall burden.

Managing Stress for Thyroid Health

Reducing stress is not just a luxury—it is a necessity for managing Hashimoto's. Practical strategies include mindfulness and meditation, which can help lower cortisol levels and improve emotional resilience. Engaging in these practices regularly fosters a sense of calm and allows you to better manage life's challenges.

Gentle exercises, such as yoga, walking, or swimming, can help reduce stress without overloading your system. Physical activity not only supports mental health but also promotes circulation and hormonal balance. To determine the right level of activity for your condition, start with short, low-intensity sessions and pay close attention to how your body responds. Avoid overly intense workouts, which may increase cortisol levels and counteract these benefits.

Prioritize 7-9 hours of restorative sleep each night. Create a calming bedtime routine and minimize screen time before bed. Sleep is a cornerstone of recovery, giving your body the chance to repair and regulate immune function. Natural supplements like ashwagandha or rhodiola may help support your adrenal glands and moderate stress responses. Always consult your doctor before starting any new supplement to ensure it aligns with your overall treatment plan.

Learning to set boundaries and say no to unnecessary commitments is essential. Allocating time for self-care is not indulgent but crucial for overall well-being. Simple acts like journaling, spending time in nature, or connecting with loved ones can make a significant difference in managing stress.

By addressing both genetic and environmental factors and learning to manage stress effectively, you can take meaningful steps to reduce the impact of Hashimoto's on your life. While you cannot change your genetics, understanding your triggers and stress responses empowers you to make choices that support your thyroid health and overall well-being. Each step you take in managing stress and identifying triggers brings you closer to a healthier, more balanced life.

Nutritional Deficiencies

Nutritional deficiencies play a pivotal role in the development and progression of Hashimoto's, as well as in the severity of its symptoms. The thyroid relies on specific nutrients to produce hormones, regulate metabolism, and maintain overall health. When these nutrients are lacking, thyroid function can decline, exacerbating symptoms such as fatigue, brain fog, hair loss, and weight gain. Understanding and addressing these deficiencies is a critical step in managing Hashimoto's effectively.

Before diving into the list of key nutrients, it's important to acknowledge that this information might feel a bit "scolastic" or technical. We could spend hours discussing each of these nutrients in detail, as their roles in thyroid health are complex and multifaceted. However, to keep our focus on the bigger picture and your immediate needs, I'll provide a concise overview. Forgive me, dear experts, for simplifying what is undoubtedly a rich and nuanced topic. Let's explore the essentials that could make a real difference in your journey toward healing.

Key Nutrients and Their Roles

Selenium

Role: Selenium is essential for the production of thyroid hormones and the protection of thyroid cells from oxidative stress. It is a key component of enzymes like glutathione peroxidase, which neutralize free radicals and reduce inflammation in the thyroid.

Impact of Deficiency: Low selenium levels can increase the risk of autoimmune activity, as the thyroid becomes more vulnerable to damage from oxidative stress. This can lead to a further decline in thyroid function.

Sources: Brazil nuts, sunflower seeds, seafood, and eggs are excellent sources of selenium. Just two Brazil nuts a day can meet your selenium needs.

Zinc

Role: Zinc supports thyroid hormone production and conversion, as well as immune system regulation. It plays a critical role in converting T4 (inactive thyroid hormone) to T3 (active thyroid hormone).

Impact of Deficiency: A zinc deficiency can impair this conversion process, leading to low T3 levels and persistent symptoms such as fatigue and poor concentration, even when T4 and TSH levels are within range.

Sources: Oysters, pumpkin seeds, chickpeas, and lean meats are rich in zinc. Adding these foods to your diet can help restore optimal thyroid function.

Vitamin D

Role: Vitamin D is crucial for modulating the immune system and reducing autoimmune activity. It helps balance the immune response, preventing it from attacking healthy thyroid tissue.

Impact of Deficiency: Low vitamin D levels are commonly found in individuals with Hashimoto's and are associated with increased inflammation and antibody levels. Without sufficient vitamin D, the autoimmune process can accelerate, worsening symptoms.

Sources: Fatty fish, fortified foods, and sunlight exposure are primary sources of vitamin D. Supplements may be necessary to reach optimal levels, particularly in individuals with limited sun exposure.

Iron

Role: Iron is vital for the production of thyroid hormones and the transport of oxygen throughout the body. It is a critical component of the enzyme thyroid peroxidase (TPO), which helps synthesize T4 and T3.

Impact of Deficiency: Iron deficiency, even in its mildest form, can impair thyroid function and lead to symptoms such as fatigue, hair thinning, and cold intolerance. In individuals with Hashimoto's, low iron levels may worsen hypothyroid symptoms.

Sources: Red meat, spinach, lentils, and fortified cereals are excellent sources of iron. Pairing iron-rich foods with vitamin C can enhance absorption.

Magnesium

Role: Magnesium is essential for energy production, nerve function, and the regulation of thyroid hormones. It also helps relax muscles and supports sleep, which are critical for overall health.

Impact of Deficiency: Magnesium deficiency can exacerbate fatigue, muscle cramps, and stress, all of which are common in Hashimoto's patients. Chronic stress further depletes magnesium levels, creating a vicious cycle.

Sources: Leafy greens, nuts, seeds, and whole grains are rich in magnesium. Supplements can also be considered under medical supervision.

Vitamin A

Role: Essential for the immune system and the regulation of the inflammatory response. It supports the conversion of T4 into T3 and protects thyroid tissue.

Impact of Deficiency: A lack of vitamin A can weaken the immune system and increase inflammation, potentially worsening Hashimoto's symptoms.

Sources: Carrots, sweet potatoes, spinach, apricots, and liver are rich in vitamin A.

Omega-3 Fatty Acids

Role: Omega-3s are known for reducing systemic inflammation and supporting immune health.

Impact of Deficiency: Low levels of omega-3 fatty acids can lead to increased inflammation, worsening autoimmune symptoms and thyroid dysfunction.

Sources: Salmon, mackerel, flaxseeds, chia seeds, and walnuts are excellent sources of omega-3s.

Iodine (With Caution)

Role: Necessary for the synthesis of T4 and T3 hormones. However, iodine must be consumed in moderation to avoid exacerbating autoimmune activity.

Impact of Deficiency: Low iodine levels can impair thyroid hormone production, while excessive intake can increase autoimmune activity.

Sources: Iodized salt, seafood, and eggs provide iodine. For individuals with Hashimoto's, iodine supplementation should be carefully monitored.

B Vitamins (B12, B6, Folate)

Role: B vitamins support energy production, metabolism, and neurological health. B12, in particular, is critical for combating fatigue and brain fog.

Impact of Deficiency: A lack of B vitamins can lead to exacerbated fatigue, poor concentration, and mood disturbances.

Sources: Meat, fish, eggs, dairy, legumes, and fortified cereals. Vegans may require B12 supplementation.

Copper

Role: Supports thyroid enzyme function and protects against oxidative stress.

Impact of Deficiency: Low copper levels can impair metabolic processes and immune response.

Sources: Sunflower seeds, nuts, liver, and dark chocolate are good sources of copper.

Probiotics and Prebiotics

Role: Promote gut health, which is critical for immune regulation and reducing systemic inflammation.

Impact of Deficiency: An imbalance in gut microbiota can contribute to leaky gut syndrome, exacerbating autoimmune conditions like Hashimoto's.

Sources: Yogurt, kefir, kimchi, and high-fiber foods such as bananas and asparagus.

Addressing Nutritional Deficiencies

To manage Hashimoto's effectively, it's essential to identify and address nutritional deficiencies through comprehensive blood testing, dietary changes, and, when necessary, supplementation. Blood tests can reveal specific deficiencies, such as low levels of selenium, vitamin D, or iron, providing a clear picture of what your body needs. Tests such as serum ferritin (for iron), 25-hydroxyvitamin D (for vitamin D), and plasma zinc levels can help pinpoint gaps that require targeted interventions.

Additionally, work with a healthcare provider or nutritionist to perform a complete thyroid panel alongside micronutrient testing. This can ensure that your dietary adjustments or supplementation are precise and effective.

Prioritize Whole Foods: Focus on nutrient-dense foods such as fresh vegetables, fruits, lean proteins, nuts, and seeds to ensure a broad spectrum of vitamins and minerals. Rotate food sources to avoid deficiencies linked to limited diets.

Cook Smart: Some nutrients, like iron and magnesium, are better absorbed when cooked, while others, like vitamin C, are sensitive to heat. For example, lightly steaming vegetables preserves their vitamin content while enhancing mineral bioavailability.

Track Progress: Retest blood levels periodically to ensure that dietary changes and supplementation are addressing deficiencies effectively.

Consider Supplements: In cases of significant deficiencies, supplements may be necessary. Work with a healthcare provider to determine appropriate dosages and ensure they align with your overall treatment plan. Always choose high-quality, third-party tested supplements to avoid fillers or contaminants.

By using testing as your guide and making informed adjustments, you can improve thyroid function, reduce inflammation, and alleviate many of the symptoms associated with Hashimoto's. Taking proactive steps empowers you to support your thyroid and take control of your health journey with confidence and clarity.

Gut Health and Autoimmunity

The connection between gut health and autoimmune conditions like Hashimoto's has become a critical focus in understanding and managing these diseases. The gut is often referred to as the "second brain" due to its profound impact on overall health, including immune system regulation. When gut health is compromised, the body's ability to distinguish between harmful invaders and its own tissues becomes impaired, leading to increased inflammation and autoimmune activity. One of the most significant contributors to this imbalance is a condition known as intestinal permeability, commonly referred to as "leaky gut."

What is Leaky Gut?

The lining of the gut acts as a barrier, selectively allowing nutrients to pass into the bloodstream while keeping harmful substances, such as toxins and undigested food particles, out. In a healthy gut, this barrier is tightly regulated. However, when the gut lining becomes compromised, gaps can form between the cells, allowing unwanted substances to leak into the bloodstream. This triggers an immune response, as the body perceives these substances as threats, leading to systemic inflammation.

In individuals with Hashimoto's, leaky gut can exacerbate autoimmune activity by creating a cycle of inflammation. As the immune system works to combat these perceived threats, it may also attack the thyroid, mistaking it for a harmful invader. This cycle perpetuates thyroid damage and worsens symptoms such as fatigue, brain fog, and joint pain.

Leaky gut can also increase the body's sensitivity to environmental and dietary triggers, such as gluten and dairy, which can further activate the immune system. Over time, this chronic inflammation can weaken the gut barrier even further, deepening the impact on overall health.

How Gut Health Impacts Autoimmunity

Microbiome Imbalance: The gut microbiome, composed of trillions of bacteria, plays a key role in regulating the immune system. A diverse and balanced microbiome supports healthy immune responses, while dysbiosis (an imbalance of gut bacteria) can lead to increased inflammation and a heightened risk of autoimmunity. Certain bacteria are particularly protective, helping to maintain the integrity of the gut lining and modulate immune activity. For instance, beneficial strains like Lactobacillus and Bifidobacterium are known to support gut health and immune balance.

Nutrient Absorption: The gut is responsible for absorbing essential nutrients like selenium, zinc, and vitamin D—all critical for thyroid health. A compromised gut lining can impair nutrient absorption, further exacerbating thyroid dysfunction and autoimmune symptoms. Additionally, chronic gut inflammation can deplete essential vitamins and minerals, even if they are present in the diet.

Systemic Inflammation: When the gut is inflamed, it can lead to the release of pro-inflammatory cytokines, signaling molecules that exacerbate systemic inflammation. This heightened inflammatory state can amplify autoimmune activity, accelerating thyroid damage. Furthermore, this systemic inflammation can contribute to symptoms such as joint pain, fatigue, and even depression, which are commonly reported by individuals with Hashimoto's.

Signs of Gut Dysfunction

Recognizing the signs of gut dysfunction is essential for identifying its role in autoimmune conditions. Symptoms often include:

- Persistent bloating or gas, particularly after meals.
- Food sensitivities or intolerances that seem to increase over time, such as to gluten, dairy, or nightshades.
- Frequent diarrhea, constipation, or alternating bowel patterns, which may signal an imbalance in the gut microbiome.
- Brain fog and fatigue, often linked to systemic inflammation originating from the gut.
- Joint pain or skin conditions, such as eczema, psoriasis, or acne, which are outward signs of internal inflammation.
- Difficulty losing weight or unexplained weight changes, often due to impaired nutrient absorption or hormonal disruptions caused by gut inflammation.

Other subtle indicators of gut dysfunction may include bad breath, frequent infections, or an increased susceptibility to colds and illnesses due to weakened immunity.

If you recognize these symptoms, it's worth investigating your gut health as a potential contributor to your Hashimoto's symptoms. Tools such as stool analysis, food sensitivity testing, and intestinal permeability assessments can provide a clearer picture of what's happening inside your gut. Left unaddressed, gut dysfunction can perpetuate the cycle of inflammation, disrupt thyroid function, and worsen autoimmune activity. Taking proactive steps to identify and address these issues can significantly improve your overall well-being and thyroid health.

Healing the Gut to Manage Autoimmunity

Adopt an Anti-Inflammatory Diet: Focus on whole, nutrient-dense foods while eliminating common inflammatory triggers such as gluten, dairy, refined sugars, and processed foods. Many individuals with Hashimoto's find relief by adopting a gluten-free or autoimmune protocol (AIP) diet. Incorporating omega-3-rich foods like salmon and flaxseeds can also help reduce inflammation.

Support the Microbiome: Include probiotic-rich foods like yogurt, kefir, sauerkraut, and kimchi to introduce beneficial bacteria. Prebiotic foods such as garlic, onions, and asparagus feed these bacteria, helping to restore balance. Probiotic supplements can be particularly useful for replenishing beneficial strains after antibiotic use or during periods of stress.

Repair the Gut Lining: Certain nutrients, such as L-glutamine, zinc, and omega-3 fatty acids, can help repair the gut lining and reduce intestinal permeability. Bone broth is another excellent option for supporting gut healing due to its high collagen content. Supplements like aloe vera or slippery elm may also soothe the gut lining and promote recovery.

Reduce Stress: Chronic stress can weaken the gut barrier and disrupt the microbiome. Incorporating mindfulness practices, such as meditation or deep breathing exercises, can significantly improve gut health. Gentle activities like yoga or tai chi can further reduce stress and support overall well-being.

Avoid Toxins: Reduce exposure to environmental toxins, such as pesticides and BPA, which can disrupt gut health. Opt for organic produce, filtered water, and BPA-free containers whenever possible. Regular detoxification practices, such as increasing fiber intake to promote elimination, can also support gut health.

Work with a Professional: A healthcare provider or functional medicine practitioner can guide you through specific testing, such as stool analysis or food sensitivity testing, to identify underlying gut issues and tailor a personalized treatment plan. Advanced tests, like intestinal permeability assessments, can provide additional insights into the health of your gut barrier.

Healing the gut is not a quick fix, but it is a foundational step in managing Hashimoto's and reducing autoimmune activity. By addressing intestinal permeability and supporting a healthy microbiome, you can break the cycle of inflammation and protect your thyroid from further damage. Over time, these interventions can enhance nutrient absorption, reduce systemic inflammation, and restore immune balance.

Small, consistent changes in your diet and lifestyle can lead to profound improvements in your overall health and well-being. Empowering yourself with knowledge and taking actionable steps to heal your gut will set the stage for long-term vitality, allowing you to take control of your Hashimoto's journey with confidence and resilience.

Hormonal Imbalances

The thyroid gland does not work in isolation. It is part of an intricate endocrine system that includes the adrenal glands, reproductive organs, and other hormonal pathways. If you've ever felt that managing Hashimoto's is overwhelming, you're not alone—many individuals face similar struggles with hormonal imbalances compounding their symptoms. Together, we'll explore how these systems interact and how to bring them back into balance, step by step. When one part of this system is out of balance, it can ripple through the body, amplifying symptoms and complicating the management of Hashimoto's. Understanding the interaction between thyroid hormones, cortisol, and sex hormones is key to breaking this cycle and restoring balance.

The Thyroid and Cortisol: The Stress Connection

Cortisol, commonly known as the stress hormone, is produced by the adrenal glands in response to physical or emotional stress. While short bursts of cortisol are beneficial, chronic stress can lead to sustained high cortisol levels, which interfere with thyroid function in several ways:

Disrupted Hormone Production: Elevated cortisol levels suppress the hypothalamic-pituitary-thyroid (HPT) axis, reducing the production of thyroid hormones. This can result in lower T3 and T4 levels, exacerbating hypothyroid symptoms such as fatigue, weight gain, and depression.

Impaired Conversion of T4 to T3: Cortisol affects the liver and other tissues responsible for converting T4 (inactive thyroid hormone) to T3 (active thyroid hormone). This can lead to a buildup of reverse T3, a form that is inactive but competes with T3 for receptor sites, further decreasing thyroid function.

Inflammatory Cascade: Chronic stress and elevated cortisol levels promote inflammation, which can worsen the autoimmune activity in Hashimoto's. Prolonged inflammation also impairs immune regulation, making it harder for the body to distinguish between healthy tissues and harmful invaders.

Adrenal Fatigue: Sustained cortisol elevation can lead to adrenal fatigue, where the adrenal glands struggle to produce sufficient cortisol. This can cause extreme fatigue, low blood pressure, and a diminished ability to handle stress, compounding Hashimoto's symptoms.

The Thyroid and Sex Hormones

The relationship between thyroid hormones and sex hormones (estrogen, progesterone, and testosterone) is equally significant. These hormones work in harmony to regulate metabolism, mood, energy levels, and reproductive health. However, an imbalance in one can disrupt the others:

Estrogen Dominance: Elevated levels of estrogen relative to progesterone, a condition known as estrogen dominance, can reduce the availability of thyroid hormones. Estrogen increases the production of thyroid-binding globulin (TBG), a protein that binds to thyroid hormones in the bloodstream, making them inactive and unavailable for cellular use. High estrogen levels can also contribute to weight gain and mood instability.

Progesterone's Protective Role: Progesterone has an anti-inflammatory effect and supports thyroid function. Low progesterone levels, often seen in women with hormonal imbalances, can increase inflammation and worsen autoimmune activity in Hashimoto's. Progesterone also plays a role in promoting restorative sleep, which is essential for thyroid health.

Testosterone and Energy Levels: Low testosterone levels, more common in men and postmenopausal women, can contribute to fatigue, muscle weakness, and reduced motivation, compounding the symptoms of hypothyroidism. Testosterone also supports bone density and muscle mass, both of which can be compromised in thyroid disorders.

Hormonal Fluctuations During Life Stages: Major life events such as pregnancy, menopause, or perimenopause can significantly impact the interplay between thyroid and sex hormones. For example, postpartum thyroiditis can trigger or exacerbate Hashimoto's, while menopause often intensifies symptoms due to declining progesterone and estrogen levels.

Signs of Hormonal Imbalances

Recognizing the signs of hormonal imbalances is the first step toward addressing them. If you've noticed these symptoms in your daily life, take heart: understanding what's happening in your body is a powerful tool for change. Common indicators include:

- Irregular menstrual cycles or heavy periods
- Fatigue and low energy levels
- Mood swings, anxiety, or depression
- Decreased libido
- Unexplained weight gain or difficulty losing weight
- Hair thinning or loss
- Poor sleep quality or insomnia
- Hot flashes or night sweats

Restoring Hormonal Balance

Manage Stress: Practice stress-reducing techniques such as mindfulness, meditation, and yoga. These activities can help regulate cortisol levels and promote a sense of calm. Aim for consistent daily practices, even if only for 10–15 minutes. Incorporating deep breathing exercises or progressive muscle relaxation can further enhance stress management. Later in this book, we dedicate an entire chapter to the topic of stress, exploring its profound impact on Hashimoto's and providing detailed strategies to manage it effectively. I encourage you to refer to that section for a deeper dive into this critical area of health.

Support the Adrenals: Nutrients like vitamin C, magnesium, and B vitamins are essential for adrenal health. Foods such as citrus fruits, leafy greens, and nuts can provide these nutrients. Herbal adaptogens like ashwagandha, rhodiola, and holy basil may also help balance cortisol levels and improve the body's resilience to stress. Staying hydrated and ensuring consistent meal timings can further support adrenal function.

Balance Estrogen and Progesterone: Focus on a diet rich in fiber, cruciferous vegetables (such as broccoli and cauliflower), and healthy fats to support estrogen metabolism and reduce estrogen dominance. Consider seed cycling, a natural method to balance hormones using flaxseeds, sesame seeds, sunflower seeds, and pumpkin seeds. Limiting alcohol and caffeine can also positively influence hormonal balance.

Promote Testosterone Levels: Engage in regular strength training exercises and ensure adequate protein intake to support muscle health and testosterone production. Foods rich in zinc, such as oysters and pumpkin seeds, can also help. Adequate sleep and reducing chronic stress are additional ways to support testosterone levels naturally.

Work with a Healthcare Professional: Hormonal imbalances can be complex, and testing is often necessary to determine specific deficiencies or excesses. Blood tests, saliva tests, or urine panels can measure cortisol patterns, estrogen, progesterone, and testosterone levels, providing a clearer picture of your hormonal health. A healthcare provider can recommend targeted interventions, such as bioidentical hormone replacement therapy (BHRT) or tailored supplementation, to address imbalances effectively.

Prioritize Restorative Sleep: Sleep is essential for hormonal regulation. Create a calming bedtime routine, minimize screen time before bed, and keep your sleeping environment cool and dark. Natural sleep aids such as magnesium glycinate or chamomile tea can support better rest.

Addressing hormonal imbalances is a vital part of managing Hashimoto's effectively. Remember, this journey is not about perfection—it's about progress. Each small step you take to balance your hormones is a victory, bringing you closer to reclaiming your health and vitality. By understanding the interconnectedness of the thyroid, cortisol, and sex hormones, you can take targeted steps to restore balance and reduce symptoms. Small, consistent changes in your diet, lifestyle, and stress management practices can have a profound impact, helping you reclaim energy, improve mood, and achieve a greater sense of well-being. Hormonal health is not just about addressing isolated issues—it's about nurturing the entire endocrine system to work in harmony. By doing so, you empower yourself to manage Hashimoto's and thrive in your daily life.

Part 2: Nutrition for Hashimoto's

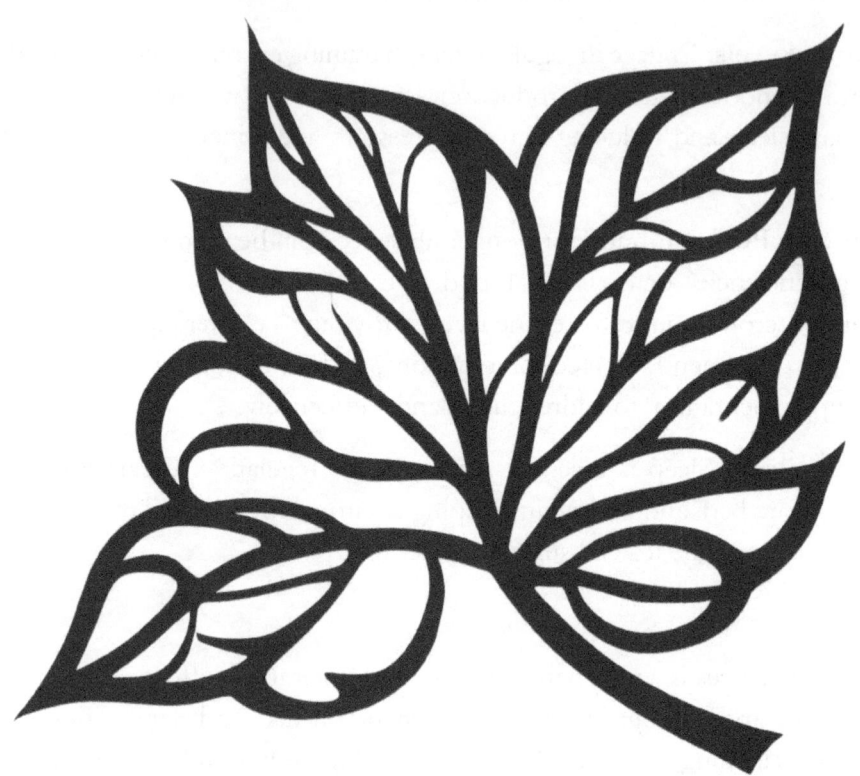

Food as Medicine

Why Diet Matters in Autoimmune Conditions

The food we consume plays a profound role in our overall health, and for those with autoimmune conditions like Hashimoto's, diet can be a transformative tool. Hashimoto's thyroiditis is not just a condition of the thyroid—it's an autoimmune disease rooted in chronic inflammation. By choosing the right foods, you can help reduce inflammation, support thyroid function, and manage symptoms more effectively.

Autoimmune diseases are characterized by the immune system attacking healthy tissue, often leading to chronic inflammation. In the case of Hashimoto's, the immune system targets the thyroid gland, impairing its ability to regulate metabolism, energy levels, and body temperature. The connection between food and inflammation is well-documented: some foods can exacerbate the immune response, while others can help soothe it. By addressing inflammation through diet, you're not only supporting your thyroid but also reducing the systemic burden on your body.

Several dietary approaches have shown promise in managing autoimmune conditions, each offering unique benefits depending on individual needs and sensitivities:

The Anti-Inflammatory Diet: Focuses on whole, unprocessed foods like fruits, vegetables, lean proteins, and healthy fats. These foods are rich in antioxidants and nutrients that combat inflammation. This diet is particularly effective in reducing the systemic burden on the body, which is crucial for managing chronic inflammation associated with autoimmune diseases.

The Paleo Diet: Eliminates grains, dairy, legumes, and processed foods, emphasizing nutrient-dense options like vegetables, nuts, seeds, and high-quality proteins. It is particularly helpful for individuals aiming to avoid potential inflammatory triggers while ensuring a rich intake of essential nutrients. The focus on whole, natural foods can help improve gut health, which is often compromised in autoimmune conditions.

The Gluten-Free Diet: Is particularly relevant for individuals with Hashimoto's. Gluten, found in wheat, barley, and rye, can trigger an immune response in some individuals, particularly those with sensitivities or celiac disease. In these cases, avoiding gluten can reduce inflammation and lessen the autoimmune attack on the thyroid, providing relief from symptoms like brain fog and fatigue.

Each person's response to these dietary approaches may vary, so it's important to experiment under the guidance of a healthcare professional to find what works best for you. Keeping a food diary can also help identify patterns and sensitivities that may not be immediately apparent. The recipes in **Part 3: The Hashimoto's Cookbook** are designed to align with these principles, offering nutrient-dense, anti-inflammatory meals that support thyroid health and overall well-being.

What to Eat

Anti-Inflammatory Foods

The foundation of a diet for Hashimoto's is built on anti-inflammatory foods. These nutrient-dense options help reduce inflammation, support immune function, and promote overall thyroid health. By incorporating a variety of fresh, whole ingredients into your meals, you can create a diet that soothes your body and minimizes autoimmune triggers. Anti-inflammatory foods are not only beneficial for managing Hashimoto's but also support overall health by reducing the risk of chronic diseases.

Vegetables: A Powerhouse of Nutrients

Leafy Greens: Spinach, kale, Swiss chard, and arugula are rich in vitamins A, C, and K, along with magnesium and iron. These nutrients enhance immune health and energy levels. Leafy greens also support liver detoxification, a critical process in managing Hashimoto's. For instance, a kale and spinach salad with olive oil dressing can be a simple yet powerful addition to your day.

Cruciferous Vegetables: Broccoli, cauliflower, and Brussels sprouts, when cooked, are safe for thyroid health despite their goitrogenic properties. These vegetables provide fiber and sulforaphane, a compound that may reduce inflammation at the cellular level and protect against oxidative damage.

Seasonal Picks: Seasonal produce like zucchini in summer or squash in autumn offers peak nutritional value. Seasonal eating ensures variety, keeps meals exciting, and maximizes nutrient intake.

Root Vegetables: Carrots, beets, and parsnips are packed with fiber, antioxidants, and natural sweetness. Roasting these vegetables with olive oil and thyme enhances their flavors, making them a nutrient-dense and satisfying side dish.

Fruits: Sweet and Functional

Berries: Blueberries, strawberries, and raspberries are packed with anthocyanins, potent antioxidants that protect thyroid cells from oxidative damage. Add them to oatmeal, sprinkle on salads, or enjoy them as a snack to boost your intake of anti-inflammatory compounds.

Citrus Fruits: Oranges, lemons, and grapefruits provide vitamin C, essential for immune health and tissue repair. A splash of lemon in your water can refresh and hydrate while boosting your vitamin intake.

Fiber-Rich Options: Apples and pears regulate digestion and stabilize blood sugar levels, supporting sustained energy. Their pectin content also promotes gut health, which is closely tied to immune function.

Exotic Fruits: Papaya and mangoes offer unique enzymes that support digestion and reduce inflammation. These can be blended into smoothies for a nutrient-packed treat.

Healthy Fats: Building Blocks for Hormonal Health

Avocado: A creamy, versatile fruit packed with monounsaturated fats and potassium. Add slices to breakfast toast or blend into a smoothie for a nutrient-dense boost. Avocados also contain glutathione, which supports liver function.

Extra Virgin Olive Oil: Rich in oleic acid, this oil has been shown to reduce inflammatory markers and enhance heart health. Use it liberally in salad dressings, drizzle over roasted vegetables, or add a tablespoon to soups for a depth of flavor.

Nuts and Seeds: Almonds, walnuts, flaxseeds, and chia seeds provide omega-3s, vitamin E, and zinc. A handful of mixed nuts can serve as a convenient, inflammation-fighting snack. Ground flaxseeds can be added to smoothies or baked goods for an extra nutrient boost.

Spices and Herbs: The Secret Weapons

Natural flavor enhancers like turmeric, ginger, cinnamon, and garlic bring both taste and therapeutic benefits. For example:

Turmeric: Contains curcumin, a compound extensively studied for its ability to lower inflammatory markers. Add a pinch to soups, teas, or even scrambled eggs.

Ginger: Aids digestion and reduces inflammation, making it an excellent addition to teas or stir-fries.

Garlic: Enhances immunity and reduces inflammation; roast it to mellow its flavor and add depth to dishes.

Tips for Choosing and Using Fresh Ingredients

Shop Locally: Farmers' markets are excellent for sourcing seasonal and nutrient-rich produce. Buying local also supports sustainability.

Go for Vibrancy: Choose vegetables and fruits that are brightly colored and firm to the touch, indicating freshness.

Prep Ahead: Wash and chop produce as soon as you bring it home to encourage frequent use. Store greens with a damp paper towel to maintain their crispness.

Experiment: Try new combinations, like roasted Brussels sprouts with a drizzle of honey or steamed spinach with garlic and lemon. Experimenting with spices like smoked paprika or fresh rosemary can elevate simple dishes.

By integrating anti-inflammatory foods into your meals, you'll not only support your thyroid but also experience better energy, digestion, and overall well-being. The recipes in Part 3 of this book will guide you in using these ingredients creatively and effectively.

Proteins, Fats, and Carbs: Finding the Right Balance

Balancing macronutrients is key to maintaining steady energy levels and reducing inflammation. For individuals with Hashimoto's, focusing on high-quality proteins, healthy fats, and complex carbohydrates can make a significant difference in managing symptoms and improving overall well-being. A balanced diet also supports hormonal regulation, digestive health, and long-term metabolic stability.

Proteins

Proteins are vital for tissue repair, muscle maintenance, and hormone production. They are especially important for stabilizing blood sugar levels, which can fluctuate in individuals with thyroid issues. Beyond their basic functions, proteins also support the immune system and help repair cellular damage caused by inflammation. Prioritize high-quality protein sources, such as:

Poultry: Chicken and turkey, preferably organic or free-range, are versatile and easy to prepare. Opt for skinless cuts to reduce saturated fat content while still benefiting from their high protein levels.

Fish: Fatty fish like salmon, mackerel, and sardines provide both protein and omega-3 fatty acids, which reduce inflammation and support cardiovascular health. These are excellent for managing systemic inflammation common in autoimmune conditions.

Plant-based options: Lentils, chickpeas, quinoa, and tofu are excellent sources of plant-based protein for those reducing animal products. They also contain fiber, which aids in gut health, a critical factor for those with Hashimoto's.

Eggs: Packed with essential amino acids and choline, eggs are a nutrient-dense protein option that also supports brain health.

Aim to include a portion of protein with every meal to stabilize blood sugar levels and maintain energy throughout the day. For example, a breakfast of scrambled eggs with spinach and a side of avocado provides protein and healthy fats to start your day right.

Healthy Fats

Healthy fats play a crucial role in reducing inflammation and supporting cognitive and hormonal health. They also improve the absorption of fat-soluble vitamins like A, D, E, and K, which are essential for overall well-being. Include fats from sources like extra-virgin olive oil, avocados, nuts, and seeds in your diet. Avoid trans fats and highly processed oils, which can contribute to inflammation.

- **Omega-3s**: Found in fish, walnuts, flaxseeds, and chia seeds, omega-3s combat systemic inflammation. They also support brain health and mood regulation, which are often affected in individuals with Hashimoto's.
- **Monounsaturated fats**: Sources like olive oil, avocados, and nuts provide energy and improve heart health. These fats also contribute to sustained energy throughout the day.
- **Cooking tips**: Adding a drizzle of olive oil over steamed vegetables, a handful of walnuts to your salad, or a slice of avocado to your morning toast are simple ways to integrate healthy fats into your meals. Another idea is blending flaxseeds into a smoothie for an added boost of omega-3s and fiber.

Carbohydrates

Carbohydrates are your body's primary source of energy. Focus on complex carbohydrates that release energy slowly, helping to regulate blood sugar levels and reduce inflammation. Avoid refined carbohydrates, such as white bread and sugary snacks, as these can cause spikes in blood sugar and contribute to fatigue and inflammation.

- **Whole grains**: Quinoa, brown rice, and oats are excellent sources of complex carbohydrates and essential minerals like magnesium and selenium.
- **Starchy vegetables**: Sweet potatoes, carrots, and parsnips offer fiber, vitamins, and natural sweetness. These can be roasted or steamed for a nutrient-rich side dish.
- **Legumes**: Black beans, lentils, and chickpeas provide both carbohydrates and protein, making them a versatile addition to meals. They are particularly beneficial for stabilizing energy levels and promoting gut health.

Pairing carbohydrates with protein and healthy fats can further stabilize blood sugar levels and enhance satiety. For example, combine roasted sweet potatoes with grilled chicken and a side of sautéed spinach for a nutrient-dense, balanced meal. Adding a small drizzle of tahini or olive oil enhances both flavor and nutritional value.

Customizing Your Balance

Everyone's nutritional needs are different, so finding the right balance of macronutrients is a personal journey. Listening to your body and working with a healthcare professional can help you determine the proportions that work best for you. For many with Hashimoto's, a diet that emphasizes protein and healthy fats while moderating carbohydrates works well to manage energy levels and inflammation. Tracking your meals and how you feel afterward can offer valuable insights into what works for your unique body.

By understanding the role of proteins, fats, and carbohydrates in your diet, you can create meals that not only nourish your body but also support your thyroid health and overall vitality. These principles will be explored in greater depth in the recipe and meal plan sections of this book, providing practical examples and guidance to help you apply them effortlessly to your daily life.

What to Avoid

Gluten, Dairy, Soy: Myths vs. Reality

For individuals with Hashimoto's, certain foods can exacerbate inflammation and trigger autoimmune responses. Gluten, dairy, and soy are often at the top of the list of potential culprits. While not everyone with Hashimoto's will need to avoid all three, understanding their potential impact can help you make informed dietary choices. By gaining clarity on why these foods might be problematic and discovering practical alternatives, you can support your thyroid health and overall well-being.

Gluten

Gluten is a protein found in wheat, barley, and rye, and it can be problematic for many individuals with Hashimoto's. Research suggests that gluten's molecular structure closely resembles that of thyroid tissue. This similarity can lead to a phenomenon known as molecular mimicry, where the immune system's attack on gluten may inadvertently target the thyroid. Additionally, gluten can increase intestinal permeability (commonly referred to as "leaky gut"), further exacerbating autoimmune activity.

For instance, Maria, a busy professional managing Hashimoto's, noticed significant improvements in her energy levels and reduced brain fog within weeks of eliminating gluten from her diet. Practical alternatives include gluten-free grains like quinoa, brown rice, millet, and certified gluten-free oats. For baking, almond flour, coconut flour, or cassava flour provide excellent substitutes while maintaining texture and flavor.

Dairy

Dairy products contain proteins like casein and whey, which can provoke immune responses in sensitive individuals. Additionally, lactose intolerance is common among those with autoimmune conditions, further complicating the digestion of dairy. Chronic consumption of dairy for those who are sensitive may lead to symptoms like bloating, skin irritation, and joint pain, which can compound the fatigue and discomfort already present with Hashimoto's.

Opting for dairy-free alternatives can make a significant difference. For example, switching to almond milk or coconut yogurt allowed Sarah, another Hashimoto's patient, to enjoy her morning smoothie without digestive discomfort. Nutritional yeast can also be used as a dairy-free cheese substitute, adding a cheesy flavor to dishes without the inflammatory impact.

Soy

Soy contains compounds called phytoestrogens, which can interfere with thyroid hormone production by mimicking estrogen in the body. While soy's effects are not universally negative, its ability to inhibit iodine absorption and potentially disrupt the conversion of T4 to T3 makes it a concern for individuals with Hashimoto's. Additionally, processed soy products like soy milk, tofu, and soy protein isolates often contain additives and are highly processed, making them less than ideal for those managing autoimmune conditions.

Instead of soy-based products, consider using almond or coconut milk, chickpeas as a protein alternative, and coconut aminos as a flavorful substitute for soy sauce. These options maintain variety in your diet without risking potential thyroid disruptions.

Importantly, it's about balance and individual experimentation. Avoiding soy entirely might not be necessary for everyone, but moderation can help minimize potential risks while keeping your diet enjoyable and diverse.

Managing Sugar and Processed Foods

Refined sugars and heavily processed foods are among the most significant contributors to chronic inflammation and poor thyroid health. These foods not only disrupt blood sugar balance but also add to the systemic burden on your immune system. Transitioning away from them can help stabilize energy levels, improve digestion, and reduce autoimmune flare-ups.

Refined sugars, commonly found in sweets, sodas, and packaged foods, cause rapid spikes and crashes in blood sugar levels. These fluctuations can exacerbate fatigue, brain fog, and mood swings. Over time, excess sugar consumption contributes to systemic inflammation, weight gain, and insulin resistance, all of which can strain thyroid function.

To manage sugar intake, consider replacing refined sugars with natural sweeteners like honey, maple syrup, or stevia. These options can be used sparingly to satisfy cravings without triggering inflammation. Whole fruits, such as berries, apples, and pears, offer a naturally sweet alternative while providing fiber and essential nutrients to stabilize blood sugar levels. Anna, a mother of two, discovered that preparing fruit salads with her kids became a fun, healthy substitute for sugary desserts.

Processed foods are equally problematic due to their high content of unhealthy fats, refined sugars, and chemical additives. Many processed products also contain hidden gluten, dairy, or soy, which can worsen autoimmune symptoms. For individuals with Hashimoto's, focusing on whole, minimally processed foods are key. Cooking at home allows you to control ingredients and avoid hidden additives. For example, meal prepping on Sundays helped Mark, a teacher with a hectic schedule, ensure he always had wholesome meals available during busy weekdays.

Transitioning away from sugar and processed foods doesn't mean you have to feel deprived. There are many ways to enjoy flavorful and satisfying meals while avoiding inflammatory ingredients. For example, homemade energy bites made from dates, nuts, and seeds can replace sugary snacks. Dressings and sauces can be easily prepared at home using olive oil, lemon juice, and fresh herbs. Gluten-free, dairy-free baked goods allow you to indulge in occasional treats without the negative impacts of processed ingredients.

By avoiding gluten, dairy, soy, refined sugars, and heavily processed foods, you can take a significant step toward reducing inflammation and managing your Hashimoto's symptoms. The recipes in Part 3 of this book are designed to make this transition seamless, offering practical and delicious alternatives that support your health and culinary creativity.

If you need a little break before diving into **Part 3**, feel free to sneak a peek at the bonuses I've put together for you. Just scan the QR code with your phone's camera.

Part 3: The Hashimoto's Cookbook

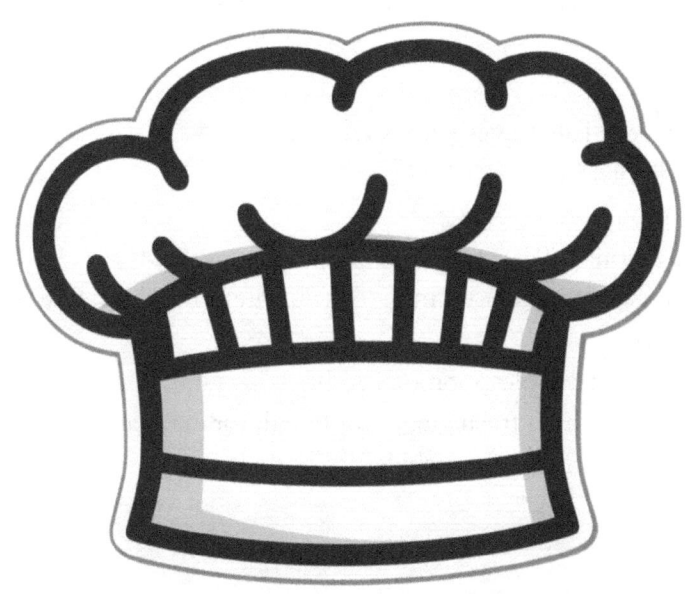

Breakfasts

Fuel Your Day with Delicious Thyroid-Friendly Recipes

Breakfast is such an important part of the day, and I'm thrilled to share some of my favorite recipes to help you start your mornings off right. In this cookbook, I've included a carefully curated selection of breakfasts that are both nourishing and thyroid-friendly.

Whether you're in the mood for a vibrant, nutrient-packed smoothie, a warm and comforting gluten-free dish, or a satisfying egg-based creation, these recipes have been crafted with care to balance flavor, nutrition, and ease. I hope they inspire you to greet each morning with a meal that energizes your body and supports your well-being.

Green Smoothie with Kale, Avocado, and Flaxseeds

This nutrient-packed green smoothie is the perfect way to start your day. Rich in omega-3s, fiber, and antioxidants, it supports thyroid health while providing a burst of energy to keep you going all morning.

Serves: 1 | **Prep Time**: 5 minutes | **Equipment Needed**: Blender, knife, cutting board | **Nutritional Information**: 250 calories, 6g protein, 18g carbohydrates, 18g fat

Ingredients:

- 1 cup (roughly 30g) fresh kale leaves (stems removed)
- 1/2 ripe avocado (about 75g)
- 1 tablespoon (10g) ground flaxseeds
- 1 small green apple (about 100g), cored and chopped
- 1/2 cup (120ml) unsweetened almond milk (or your preferred dairy-free milk)
- 1/2 cup (120ml) water
- Juice of 1/2 lemon (about 1 tablespoon or 15ml)
- 1/2 teaspoon (about 1g) grated fresh ginger (optional, for extra anti-inflammatory benefits)
- A handful of ice cubes (optional, for a chilled smoothie)

Instructions:

1. Add the kale, avocado, flaxseeds, apple, almond milk, and water to a blender.
2. Squeeze in the lemon juice and add the grated ginger, if using.
3. Blend on high speed until smooth and creamy. If the smoothie is too thick, add a little more water to reach your desired consistency.
4. Taste and adjust as needed. If you prefer a sweeter flavor, add a small piece of banana or a drizzle of honey (optional).
5. Pour into a glass, add ice cubes if desired, and enjoy immediately.

Chef's Tip:

- For a protein boost, add a scoop of unflavored or vanilla plant-based protein powder.
- To make it meal-prep friendly, prepare and freeze the ingredients (except the liquid) in individual bags for easy blending during busy mornings.

Thyroid Health Note:

This smoothie is packed with nutrients that support thyroid function. Kale provides antioxidants and vitamins, while avocado and flaxseeds deliver healthy fats and omega-3s that help reduce inflammation. Lemon juice and ginger add a refreshing anti-inflammatory kick, making this a perfect addition to your Hashimoto's-friendly diet.

Tropical Smoothie with Pineapple, Ginger, and Coconut Milk

Transport yourself to a tropical paradise with this creamy, refreshing smoothie. Packed with anti-inflammatory ingredients and thyroid-supporting nutrients, it's perfect for a morning boost or a mid-day pick-me-up.

Serves: 1 | **Prep Time**: 5 minutes | **Equipment Needed**: Blender, knife, cutting board | **Nutritional Information**: 230 calories, 2g protein, 27g carbohydrates, 14g fat

Ingredients:

- 1 cup (about 165g) fresh pineapple chunks
- 1/2 frozen banana (about 50g)
- 1/2 cup (120ml) unsweetened coconut milk
- 1/4 cup (60ml) water
- 1/2 teaspoon (about 1g) grated fresh ginger
- Juice of 1/2 lime (about 1 tablespoon or 15ml)
- 1 tablespoon (7g) shredded unsweetened coconut (optional, for garnish)
- A handful of ice cubes (optional, for a chilled smoothie)

Instructions:

- Add the pineapple, frozen banana, coconut milk, water, ginger, and lime juice to a blender.
- Blend on high speed until smooth and creamy. If the smoothie is too thick, add more water to adjust the consistency.
- Taste and adjust as needed. For a sweeter flavor, add a drizzle of honey or a small piece of additional banana.
- Pour into a glass, garnish with shredded coconut if desired, and enjoy immediately.

Chef's Tip:

- To save time, pre-portion the pineapple chunks and banana into freezer bags for quick and easy meal prep. If you want to make the smoothie more refreshing, consider adding a small handful of fresh mint leaves before blending.

Thyroid Health Note:

This tropical smoothie is rich in nutrients that support thyroid function and reduce inflammation. Pineapple contains bromelain, a natural enzyme with anti-inflammatory properties, while coconut milk provides healthy fats that support hormone production. Ginger and lime add a refreshing burst of flavor and further enhance the smoothie's anti-inflammatory benefits.

Protein Smoothie with Almond Butter and Blueberries

This creamy, protein-packed smoothie is perfect for a post-workout recovery or a nutritious start to your day. Bursting with antioxidants from blueberries and healthy fats from almond butter, it's a delicious way to support your energy and thyroid health.

Serves: 1 | **Prep Time**: 5 minutes | **Equipment Needed**: Blender, knife, measuring cups | **Nutritional Information**: 290 calories, 12g protein, 22g carbohydrates, 18g fat

Ingredients:

- 1/2 cup (75g) fresh or frozen blueberries
- 1 tablespoon (16g) almond butter
- 1/2 frozen banana (about 50g)
- 1 scoop (30g) unflavored or vanilla protein powder
- 1/2 cup (120ml) unsweetened almond milk
- 1/4 cup (60ml) water
- A handful of ice cubes (optional, for a chilled smoothie)
- 1 teaspoon (5g) chia seeds (optional, for garnish)

Instructions:

1. Add the blueberries, almond butter, banana, protein powder, almond milk, and water to a blender.
2. Blend on high speed until smooth and creamy. If the consistency is too thick, add a little more water or almond milk.
3. Taste and adjust as needed. For extra sweetness, add a drizzle of honey or a small date.
4. Pour into a glass, top with chia seeds if desired, and enjoy immediately.

Chef's Tip:

- Adding a pinch of cinnamon can enhance the flavor and provide additional anti-inflammatory benefits.

Thyroid Health Note:

This smoothie is rich in antioxidants, healthy fats, and protein—key components for thyroid support. Blueberries are loaded with antioxidants that reduce oxidative stress, while almond butter provides vitamin E and magnesium, which promote hormonal balance. The addition of protein powder ensures sustained energy and muscle recovery, making this smoothie an excellent choice for anyone managing Hashimoto's or seeking a nutrient-dense snack.

Almond Flour Pancakes with Natural Maple Syrup

These light and fluffy almond flour pancakes are a delicious gluten-free alternative to traditional pancakes. Perfect for breakfast or brunch, they're packed with protein and healthy fats to keep you energized throughout the day. Drizzle with natural maple syrup for a touch of sweetness.

Serves: 2 | **Prep Time**: 10 minutes | **Cook Time**: 15 minutes | **Equipment Needed**: Mixing bowl, whisk, non-stick skillet, spatula | **Nutritional Information**: 280 calories (per serving), 8g protein, 10g carbohydrates, 22g fat

Ingredients:

- 1 cup (100g) almond flour
- 2 large eggs
- 1/4 cup (60ml) unsweetened almond milk
- 1 tablespoon (15ml) natural maple syrup (plus extra for serving)
- 1/2 teaspoon (2g) baking powder
- 1/4 teaspoon (1g) vanilla extract
- A pinch of salt
- Coconut oil or butter for greasing the skillet

Instructions:

1. In a mixing bowl, whisk together the almond flour, baking powder, and salt.
2. In a separate bowl, beat the eggs, almond milk, maple syrup, and vanilla extract until well combined.
3. Gradually add the wet ingredients to the dry ingredients, stirring until a smooth batter forms. If the batter is too thick, add a splash more almond milk.
4. Heat a non-stick skillet over medium heat and lightly grease with coconut oil or butter.
5. Pour 2-3 tablespoons of batter onto the skillet for each pancake, spreading slightly to form a circle.
6. Cook for 2-3 minutes, or until bubbles form on the surface and the edges look set. Flip and cook for an additional 2 minutes until golden brown.
7. Repeat with the remaining batter, greasing the skillet as needed.
8. Serve warm with a drizzle of natural maple syrup and your favorite toppings, such as fresh berries or a sprinkle of cinnamon.

Chef's Tip:

- To make these pancakes extra fluffy, let the batter rest for 5 minutes before cooking.
- For added flavor, mix in a pinch of ground cinnamon or nutmeg.

Thyroid Health Note: These pancakes are a great gluten-free breakfast option that supports thyroid health. Almond flour is rich in vitamin E and magnesium, which help reduce inflammation and support hormonal balance. Using natural maple syrup as a sweetener keeps the glycemic impact lower than refined sugars, making this recipe a wholesome start to your day.

Coconut Flour Waffles with Fresh Berries

Crispy on the outside and fluffy on the inside, these coconut flour waffles are a delightful gluten-free breakfast option. Paired with fresh berries, they make for a wholesome, nutrient-packed start to your day.

Serves: 2 | **Prep Time**: 10 minutes | **Cook Time**: 15 minutes | **Equipment Needed**: Mixing bowl, whisk, waffle iron, measuring cups and spoons | **Nutritional Information**: 300 calories (per serving), 10g protein, 15g carbohydrates, 22g fat

Ingredients:

- 1/4 cup (30g) coconut flour
- 3 large eggs
- 1/4 cup (60ml) unsweetened coconut milk
- 1 tablespoon (15ml) melted coconut oil (plus extra for greasing)
- 1/2 teaspoon (2g) baking powder
- 1 teaspoon (5g) vanilla extract
- 1 tablespoon (15ml) natural maple syrup (optional, for sweetness)
- A pinch of salt
- 1/2 cup (75g) mixed fresh berries (e.g., strawberries, blueberries, raspberries) for topping

Instructions:

1. Preheat your waffle iron and lightly grease it with coconut oil.
2. In a mixing bowl, whisk together the coconut flour, baking powder, and salt.
3. In a separate bowl, beat the eggs, coconut milk, melted coconut oil, vanilla extract, and maple syrup (if using) until well combined.
4. Gradually add the wet ingredients to the dry ingredients, mixing until a smooth batter forms. Let the batter rest for 5 minutes to thicken.
5. Pour the batter into the preheated waffle iron, spreading it evenly. Cook according to your waffle iron's instructions, typically 3-5 minutes, until golden and crisp.
6. Carefully remove the waffles and repeat with the remaining batter, greasing the waffle iron as needed.
7. Serve the waffles warm, topped with fresh berries and a drizzle of maple syrup or a dusting of powdered coconut sugar, if desired.

Chef's Tip:

- To enhance the flavor, add a teaspoon of grated lemon zest to the batter.
- For a protein boost, serve with a dollop of Greek yogurt or a sprinkle of chia seeds on top.

Thyroid Health Note: These waffles are a fantastic gluten-free option that supports thyroid health. Coconut flour is high in fiber and low in carbohydrates, helping to maintain stable blood sugar levels. The fresh berries provide antioxidants that combat oxidative stress, while the healthy fats in coconut milk and oil support hormone production and reduce inflammation.

Oatmeal Bowl with Chia Seeds and Cinnamon

Warm, comforting, and packed with nutrients, this oatmeal bowl is a great way to start your day. With the addition of chia seeds for extra fiber and cinnamon for its anti-inflammatory properties, this recipe is perfect for sustained energy and supporting thyroid health.

Serves: 1 | **Prep Time**: 5 minutes | **Cook Time**: 5 minutes | **Equipment Needed**: Small saucepan, mixing spoon, measuring cups | **Nutritional Information**: 280 calories, 8g protein, 45g carbohydrates, 8g fat

Ingredients:

- 1/2 cup (50g) gluten-free rolled oats
- 1 cup (240ml) unsweetened almond milk (or water)
- 1 tablespoon (10g) chia seeds
- 1/2 teaspoon (1g) ground cinnamon
- 1 teaspoon (5ml) honey or maple syrup (optional, for sweetness)
- 1/4 cup (40g) fresh berries (e.g., blueberries, strawberries)
- 1 tablespoon (10g) chopped nuts (e.g., almonds, walnuts) for topping

Instructions:

1. In a small saucepan, combine the oats, almond milk, and chia seeds. Cook over medium heat, stirring frequently, for 3-5 minutes, or until the oats are tender and the mixture has thickened.
2. Stir in the ground cinnamon and honey or maple syrup, if using.
3. Transfer the oatmeal to a bowl and top with fresh berries and chopped nuts.
4. Serve warm and enjoy immediately.

Chef's Tip:

- For a creamier texture, cook the oats with half almond milk and half water.

Thyroid Health Note:

This oatmeal bowl is an excellent source of fiber, which supports healthy digestion and stable blood sugar levels. Chia seeds provide omega-3s and essential minerals, while cinnamon helps reduce inflammation. The combination of oats and nuts delivers sustained energy, making this a thyroid-friendly breakfast option.

Spinach, Avocado, and Sun-Dried Tomato Frittata

This delicious and nutrient-packed frittata is perfect for breakfast, brunch, or even a light dinner. Loaded with spinach, creamy avocado, and tangy sun-dried tomatoes, it's a gluten-free, high-protein option that supports thyroid health.

Serves: 2-3 | **Prep Time**: 10 minutes | **Cook Time**: 15 minutes | **Equipment Needed**: Mixing bowl, whisk, non-stick skillet, spatula, oven | **Nutritional Information**: 320 calories (per serving), 14g protein, 12g carbohydrates, 24g fat

Ingredients:

- 6 large eggs
- 1 cup (30g) fresh spinach, chopped
- 1/4 cup (40g) sun-dried tomatoes, chopped
- 1/4 teaspoon (1g) salt
- 1/2 teaspoon (1g) dried oregano (optional)
- 1/4 cup (60ml) unsweetened almond milk
- 1/2 avocado (about 75g), diced
- 1 tablespoon (15ml) olive oil (plus extra for greasing, if needed)
- 1/4 teaspoon (1g) black pepper

Instructions:

1. Preheat your oven to 375°F (190°C) if finishing the frittata in the oven, or set the stovetop to medium heat.
2. In a mixing bowl, whisk together the eggs, almond milk, salt, pepper, and oregano until well combined.
3. Heat the olive oil in a non-stick skillet over medium heat. Add the spinach and sun-dried tomatoes, cooking for
4. 2-3 minutes until the spinach is wilted.
5. Pour the egg mixture into the skillet, ensuring it evenly coats the spinach and tomatoes. Gently stir to distribute the ingredients.
6. Cook on the stovetop for 5-7 minutes, or until the edges begin to set. Add the diced avocado on top.
7. Transfer the skillet to the oven and bake for 7-10 minutes, or until the frittata is fully set and lightly golden on top. If not using an oven, continue cooking on low heat with a lid on until fully set.
8. Remove from heat, slice into wedges, and serve warm. Pair with a side salad or gluten-free toast for a complete meal.

Chef's Tip:

- For added flavor, sprinkle a handful of grated dairy-free cheese on top before baking.

Thyroid Health Note: Spinach provides vital antioxidants and magnesium, while avocado delivers healthy fats essential for hormone production. Sun-dried tomatoes add a rich source of potassium and antioxidants, supporting overall energy and reducing inflammation.

Scrambled Eggs with Mushrooms and Caramelized Onions

Soft, creamy scrambled eggs paired with earthy mushrooms and sweet caramelized onions make for a satisfying and nutrient-dense breakfast. This recipe is quick to prepare and packed with protein, making it a perfect start to your day.

Serves: 2 | **Prep Time**: 10 minutes | **Cook Time**: 15 minutes | **Equipment Needed**: Non-stick skillet, spatula, knife, cutting board | **Nutritional Information**: 250 calories (per serving), 14g protein, 10g carbohydrates, 18g fat

Ingredients:

- 4 large eggs
- 1 cup (100g) mushrooms, sliced
- 1 tablespoon (15ml) olive oil
- 1/4 teaspoon (1g) black pepper
- 1/4 cup (60ml) unsweetened almond milk
- 1/2 cup (80g) yellow onion, thinly sliced
- 1/2 teaspoon (1g) salt
- Fresh parsley or chives (optional, for garnish)

Instructions:

1. Heat 1/2 tablespoon of olive oil in a non-stick skillet over medium heat. Add the sliced onions and cook, stirring occasionally, for 8-10 minutes until they are soft and golden brown. Remove from the skillet and set aside.
2. In the same skillet, add the remaining olive oil and the mushrooms. Cook for 5 minutes, stirring occasionally, until the mushrooms are tender and lightly browned. Remove from the skillet and set aside with the onions.
3. In a mixing bowl, whisk together the eggs, almond milk, salt, and pepper until well combined.
4. Reduce the skillet heat to low and pour in the egg mixture. Stir gently with a spatula, cooking slowly until the eggs are soft and creamy, about 3-5 minutes.
5. Add the caramelized onions and mushrooms back into the skillet, folding them gently into the eggs. Cook for an additional 1-2 minutes until warmed through.
6. Serve immediately, garnished with fresh parsley or chives if desired.

Chef's Tip:

- For an extra boost of flavor, add a dash of smoked paprika.
- Pair this dish with gluten-free toast or a side of fresh greens for a complete meal.

Thyroid Health Note: This dish is rich in protein and antioxidants, supporting muscle recovery and reducing inflammation. Mushrooms provide selenium, an essential mineral for thyroid function, while onions offer natural compounds that promote immune health. Eggs are an excellent source of iodine and choline, crucial for thyroid hormone production and overall well-being.

Sweet Potato Toast with Hummus and Avocado

A nutrient-dense alternative to traditional toast, this sweet potato toast is topped with creamy hummus and avocado for a flavorful, gluten-free breakfast or snack. Packed with vitamins, healthy fats, and plant-based protein, it's a great option for supporting thyroid health and boosting energy levels.

Serves: 2 | **Prep Time**: 10 minutes | **Cook Time**: 20 minutes | **Equipment Needed**: Baking sheet, knife, cutting board, toaster or oven | **Nutritional Information**: 290 calories (per serving), 7g protein, 30g carbohydrates, 15g fat

Ingredients:

- 1 large sweet potato (about 250g), sliced lengthwise into 1/4-inch (0.6cm) thick slices
- 1/2 cup (120g) hummus
- 1 avocado (about 150g), sliced
- 1 tablespoon (15ml) olive oil
- 1/4 teaspoon (1g) salt
- 1/4 teaspoon (1g) black pepper
- Optional toppings: cherry tomatoes, red pepper flakes, fresh herbs (e.g., parsley or cilantro)

Instructions:

1. Preheat your oven to 400°F (200°C) and line a baking sheet with parchment paper.
2. Brush both sides of the sweet potato slices with olive oil and sprinkle with salt and pepper.
3. Arrange the slices in a single layer on the prepared baking sheet. Bake for 15-20 minutes, flipping halfway through, until tender and lightly browned. Alternatively, toast the sweet potato slices in a toaster on high for 3-5 minutes until cooked through.
4. Spread hummus evenly over each slice of sweet potato.
5. Top with avocado slices and your choice of optional toppings, such as cherry tomatoes, red pepper flakes, or fresh herbs.
6. Serve immediately and enjoy!

Chef's Tip:

- For a protein boost, add a sprinkle of hemp seeds or a drizzle of tahini on top.
- To save time, bake a large batch of sweet potato slices and store them in the fridge for up to 3 days. Simply reheat in a toaster or oven before serving.

Thyroid Health Note: This recipe is loaded with thyroid-supporting nutrients. Sweet potatoes provide complex carbohydrates and vitamin A, essential for energy and immune function. Avocado delivers healthy fats to support hormone production, while hummus offers plant-based protein and fiber to promote stable blood sugar levels and reduce inflammation.

Lunches and Dinners

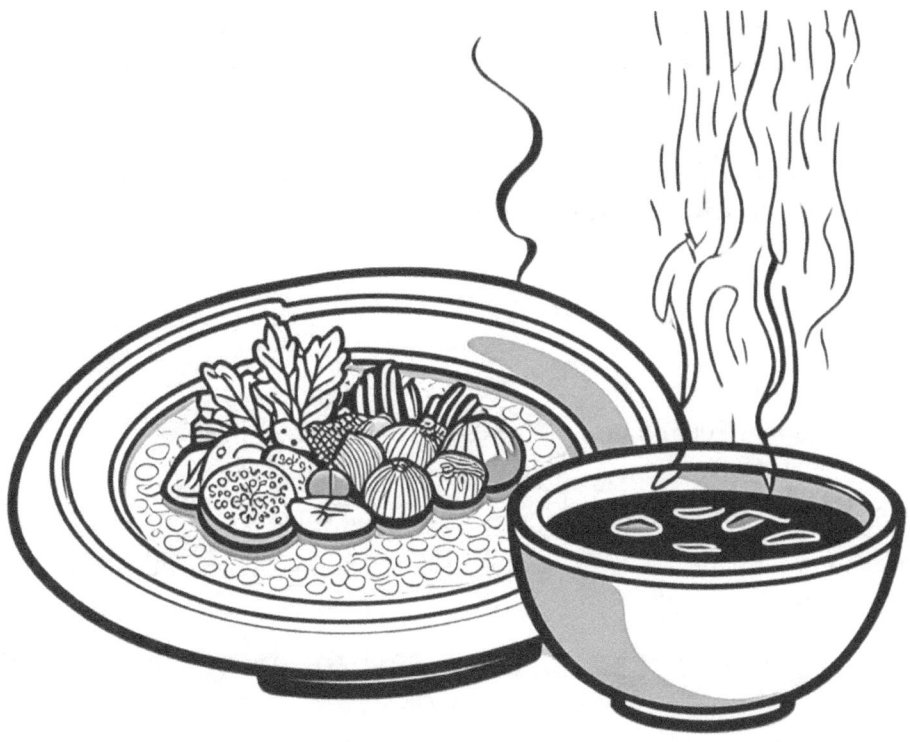

Nourishing Meals for Every Occasion

When it comes to lunches and dinners, I've put together a collection of recipes that truly celebrates variety and balance. These meals are designed to be as nourishing as they are delicious, with options to suit every craving and dietary need. Whether you're looking for something quick and easy or a dish to impress, this section has you covered with a thoughtfully curated selection of recipes.

You'll discover hearty Soups & Stews that bring comfort to your table, protein-packed bowls to keep your energy levels steady throughout the day, and simple yet flavorful Baked and One-Pan Meals that minimize prep and cleanup. For those seeking more plant-forward options, I've included creative Plant-Based Mains that deliver incredible flavor while remaining entirely meat-free. If you're focusing on reducing carbs, you'll appreciate the satisfying Low Carb Dinners that are both healthy and indulgent. And for those who love exploring global cuisine, the dishes inspired by International Flavors will take your taste buds on a journey around the world.

Each recipe in this section is crafted to support your thyroid health while ensuring you never have to compromise on taste or variety. From vibrant ingredients to simple techniques, these meals are meant to inspire confidence in your cooking and provide a sense of joy in every bite. Let this collection transform your lunch and dinner routines into opportunities for nourishment, discovery, and delight.

Red Lentil Curry Soup with Coconut Milk

This creamy, flavorful red lentil curry soup is a comforting and nutrient-rich dish perfect for lunch or dinner. Packed with plant-based protein and anti-inflammatory ingredients, it's both satisfying and supportive of thyroid health.

Serves: 4 | **Prep Time**: 10 minutes | **Cook Time**: 25 minutes | **Equipment Needed**: Large pot, wooden spoon, knife, cutting board | **Nutritional Information**: 320 calories (per serving), 12g protein, 30g carbohydrates, 15g fat

Ingredients:

- 1 cup (200g) red lentils, rinsed
- 1 small yellow onion (about 100g), finely chopped
- 1 tablespoon (15g) grated fresh ginger
- 1 teaspoon (2g) ground turmeric
- 1 can (400ml) full-fat coconut milk
- 1 medium carrot (about 80g), diced
- 1/2 teaspoon (1g) salt (or to taste)
- Juice of 1/2 lime (about 1 tablespoon or 15ml)
- 1 tablespoon (15ml) coconut oil
- 2 garlic cloves, minced
- 2 teaspoons (4g) curry powder
- 1/2 teaspoon (1g) ground cumin
- 3 cups (720ml) vegetable broth
- 1 small red bell pepper (about 100g), diced
- 1/4 teaspoon (1g) black pepper
- Fresh cilantro or parsley for garnish (optional)

Instructions:

1. Heat the coconut oil in a large pot over medium heat. Add the onion and cook for 3-4 minutes until softened.
2. Stir in the garlic, ginger, curry powder, turmeric, and cumin. Cook for 1-2 minutes, stirring frequently, until fragrant.
3. Add the red lentils, coconut milk, vegetable broth, carrot, red bell pepper, salt, and black pepper. Stir to combine.
4. Bring the mixture to a boil, then reduce the heat to low and let it simmer for 20 minutes, or until the lentils are tender and the soup has thickened.
5. Stir in the lime juice and adjust the seasoning if needed.
6. Serve hot, garnished with fresh cilantro or parsley if desired.

Chef's Tip:

- For extra protein, add a handful of cooked chickpeas to the soup before serving.

Thyroid Health Note: This soup is rich in anti-inflammatory spices like turmeric and ginger, which support immune function and reduce oxidative stress. Red lentils provide plant-based protein and iron, essential for energy production, while coconut milk delivers healthy fats that support hormone regulation and overall thyroid health.

Seasonal Vegetable Minestrone with Bone Broth

A hearty and nutrient-dense take on a classic dish, this seasonal vegetable minestrone with bone broth is packed with vitamins, minerals, and antioxidants. Perfect for a cozy meal, it supports gut health and boosts energy, making it ideal for those managing Hashimoto's.

Serves: 4-6 | **Prep Time**: 15 minutes | **Cook Time**: 30 minutes | **Equipment Needed**: Large pot, wooden spoon, knife, cutting board | **Nutritional Information**: 200 calories (per serving), 10g protein, 18g carbohydrates, 8g fat

Ingredients:

- 1 tablespoon (15ml) olive oil
- 2 garlic cloves, minced
- 2 celery stalks (about 100g), diced
- 1 cup (150g) green beans, trimmed and cut into 1-inch pieces
- 2 cups (480ml) water
- 1/2 teaspoon (1g) dried thyme
- 1/4 teaspoon (1g) black pepper
- 1/2 cup (100g) cooked cannellini beans (optional, for added protein)
- 1 small yellow onion (about 100g), finely chopped
- 2 medium carrots (about 150g), diced
- 1 medium zucchini (about 200g), diced
- 4 cups (960ml) bone broth (chicken or beef)
- 1 can (400g) diced tomatoes
- 1/2 teaspoon (1g) dried oregano
- 1/2 teaspoon (2g) salt (or to taste)
- 1/4 cup (15g) fresh parsley, chopped (optional, for garnish)

Instructions:

1. Heat the olive oil in a large pot over medium heat. Add the onion, garlic, carrots, and celery. Cook for 5-7 minutes, stirring occasionally, until the vegetables are softened.
2. Stir in the zucchini and green beans. Cook for an additional 3-4 minutes.
3. Add the bone broth, water, diced tomatoes, thyme, oregano, salt, and pepper. Bring the mixture to a boil, then reduce the heat to low and let it simmer for 20 minutes.
4. If using cannellini beans, stir them into the soup during the last 5 minutes of cooking.
5. Taste and adjust seasoning as needed. Serve hot, garnished with fresh parsley if desired.

Chef's Tip:

- For a heartier meal, add 1/2 cup (85g) of gluten-free pasta or cooked quinoa during the last 10 minutes of cooking.

Thyroid Health Note: Bone broth is rich in collagen and amino acids that support gut health and reduce inflammation, both crucial for managing Hashimoto's. The variety of vegetables provides antioxidants and fiber, supporting digestion and overall wellness. Adding cannellini beans boosts protein content, ensuring sustained energy and satiety.

Baked Chicken and Vegetable Stew

This hearty baked chicken and vegetable stew is a comforting one-pot meal, perfect for any time of year. Packed with protein, fiber, and antioxidants, it's a simple and nourishing option that supports thyroid health and keeps you energized.

Serves: 4 | **Prep Time**: 15 minutes | **Cook Time**: 1 hour | **Equipment Needed**: Baking dish with lid or foil, knife, cutting board, mixing bowl | **Nutritional Information**: 350 calories (per serving), 28g protein, 20g carbohydrates, 15g fat

Ingredients:

- 4 bone-in chicken thighs (about 600g), skin removed
- 2 celery stalks (about 100g), chopped
- 2 medium potatoes (about 300g), peeled and cubed
- 3 garlic cloves, minced
- 2 cups (480ml) chicken bone broth
- 1 teaspoon (2g) dried rosemary
- 1/2 teaspoon (1g) salt
- Fresh parsley for garnish (optional)
- 2 medium carrots (about 150g), sliced into rounds
- 1 medium onion (about 100g), diced
- 1 cup (150g) cherry tomatoes, halved
- 1 tablespoon (15ml) olive oil
- 1 teaspoon (2g) dried thyme
- 1/2 teaspoon (1g) paprika
- 1/4 teaspoon (1g) black pepper

Instructions:

1. Preheat your oven to 375°F (190°C).
2. In a large mixing bowl, combine the carrots, celery, onion, potatoes, cherry tomatoes, and garlic. Drizzle with olive oil and sprinkle with thyme, rosemary, paprika, salt, and pepper. Toss to coat evenly.
3. Transfer the vegetable mixture to a baking dish. Arrange the chicken thighs on top of the vegetables.
4. Pour the chicken bone broth over the vegetables and chicken, ensuring everything is evenly moistened.
5. Cover the baking dish with a lid or foil and bake for 45 minutes.
6. Remove the cover and bake for an additional 15 minutes to allow the chicken to brown slightly.
7. Remove from the oven, garnish with fresh parsley if desired, and serve warm. Pair with a side of gluten-free bread or steamed greens for a complete meal.

Chef's Tip:

- For extra flavor, marinate the chicken in olive oil, garlic, and herbs for 1 hour before cooking.

Thyroid Health Note: This dish is rich in protein and essential nutrients. Chicken provides lean protein for muscle repair and sustained energy, while the variety of vegetables offers antioxidants and fiber to support digestion and reduce inflammation. The bone broth adds collagen and amino acids, promoting gut health and overall thyroid function.

Slow-Cooked Beef Pot Roast with Root Vegetables

This tender and flavorful slow-cooked beef pot roast is a comforting dish perfect for family dinners or meal prep. Packed with protein and nutrient-dense root vegetables, it's a thyroid-friendly option that is both satisfying and nourishing.

Serves: 4-6 | **Prep Time**: 15 minutes | **Cook Time**: 6-8 hours (slow cooker) | **Equipment Needed**: Slow cooker or Dutch oven, knife, cutting board | **Nutritional Information**: 400 calories (per serving), 35g protein, 20g carbohydrates, 18g fat

Ingredients:

- 2 pounds (900g) beef chuck roast
- 2 medium carrots (about 150g), cut into chunks
- 1 medium yellow onion (about 100g), diced
- 2 medium potatoes (about 300g), cubed
- 1 tablespoon (15ml) tomato paste
- 1 teaspoon (2g) dried rosemary
- 1/2 teaspoon (1g) salt
- 1 bay leaf
- 1 tablespoon (15ml) olive oil
- 2 parsnips (about 150g), cut into chunks
- 3 garlic cloves, minced
- 2 cups (480ml) beef bone broth
- 1 teaspoon (2g) dried thyme
- 1/2 teaspoon (1g) paprika
- 1/4 teaspoon (1g) black pepper
- Fresh parsley for garnish (optional)

Instructions:

1. Heat the olive oil in a large skillet over medium-high heat. Sear the beef on all sides until browned, about 2-3 minutes per side. Transfer the beef to the slow cooker or Dutch oven.
2. Add the carrots, parsnips, potatoes, onion, and garlic around the beef.
3. In a small bowl, whisk together the bone broth, tomato paste, thyme, rosemary, paprika, salt, and pepper. Pour the mixture over the beef and vegetables. Add the bay leaf.
4. Cover and cook on low heat for 6-8 hours (or 3-4 hours on high), until the beef is tender and easily pulls apart with a fork.
5. Remove the bay leaf and discard. Shred the beef or slice it into portions. Taste the broth and adjust seasoning if needed.
6. Serve the pot roast with the vegetables and garnish with fresh parsley if desired.

Chef's Tip:

- For a richer flavor, deglaze the skillet with 1/4 cup (60ml) red wine after searing the beef and pour it into the slow cooker.

Thyroid Health Note: Beef provides iron and zinc, crucial for energy production and immune function, while the root vegetables offer fiber and antioxidants to support digestion and reduce inflammation. Bone broth adds collagen and amino acids, promoting gut health and thyroid function.

Quinoa Bowl with Grilled Salmon and Lemon Asparagus

This vibrant quinoa bowl features tender grilled salmon and zesty lemon asparagus, making it a protein-packed and nutrient-rich meal. Perfect for lunch or dinner, it's a flavorful way to support thyroid health and overall well-being.

Serves: 2 | **Prep Time**: 10 minutes | **Cook Time**: 20 minutes | **Equipment Needed**: Medium saucepan, grill pan or skillet, knife, cutting board | **Nutritional Information**: 450 calories (per serving), 30g protein, 28g carbohydrates, 20g fat

Ingredients:

- 1/2 cup (90g) quinoa, rinsed
- 1 cup (240ml) water or vegetable broth
- 2 salmon fillets (about 300g total)
- 1 tablespoon (15ml) olive oil, divided
- 1 bunch (200g) asparagus, trimmed
- Juice and zest of 1/2 lemon (about 1 tablespoon or 15ml juice)
- 1/2 teaspoon (1g) salt
- 1/4 teaspoon (1g) black pepper
- 1 tablespoon (4g) fresh dill, chopped (optional, for garnish)

Instructions:

1. In a medium saucepan, combine the quinoa and water or vegetable broth. Bring to a boil, then reduce the heat to low, cover, and simmer for 15 minutes or until the quinoa is tender and the liquid is absorbed. Fluff with a fork and set aside.
2. While the quinoa cooks, heat a grill pan or skillet over medium-high heat. Brush the salmon fillets with 1/2 tablespoon of olive oil and season with salt and pepper. Grill for 3-4 minutes per side, or until cooked through.
3. Toss the asparagus with the remaining olive oil, lemon juice, and zest. Grill or sauté for 5-7 minutes until tender but crisp.
4. Divide the quinoa between two bowls. Top with the grilled salmon and lemon asparagus. Garnish with fresh dill if desired and serve immediately.

Chef's Tip:

- For extra flavor, marinate the salmon in a mixture of olive oil, garlic, and lemon juice for 30 minutes before cooking.
- To save time, cook the quinoa in advance and store it in the fridge for up to 3 days.

Thyroid Health Note: This dish is rich in omega-3s from the salmon, which help reduce inflammation and support brain and thyroid function. Quinoa provides plant-based protein and essential minerals, while asparagus offers antioxidants and fiber to promote digestion and overall health.

Roasted Chicken Salad with Avocado and Sunflower Seeds

This roasted chicken salad combines creamy avocado, crunchy sunflower seeds, and a mix of fresh greens for a delicious and balanced meal. High in protein and healthy fats, it's perfect for supporting energy levels and reducing inflammation.

Serves: 2 | **Prep Time**: 10 minutes | **Cook Time**: 25 minutes | **Equipment Needed**: Baking sheet, mixing bowl, knife, cutting board | **Nutritional Information**: 400 calories (per serving), 35g protein, 12g carbohydrates, 20g fat

Ingredients:

- 2 boneless, skinless chicken breasts (about 300g total)
- 1 tablespoon (15ml) olive oil
- 1/2 teaspoon (1g) salt
- 1/4 teaspoon (1g) black pepper
- 4 cups (120g) mixed greens (e.g., spinach, arugula, kale)
- 1 avocado (about 150g), sliced
- 2 tablespoons (20g) sunflower seeds
- Juice of 1/2 lemon (about 1 tablespoon or 15ml)
- 1 tablespoon (15ml) olive oil (for dressing)
- 1 teaspoon (5ml) Dijon mustard

Instructions:

1. Preheat your oven to 400°F (200°C). Line a baking sheet with parchment paper.
2. Rub the chicken breasts with olive oil, salt, and pepper. Place them on the prepared baking sheet and roast for 20-25 minutes, or until the internal temperature reaches 165°F (74°C). Let rest for 5 minutes before slicing.
3. In a small bowl, whisk together the lemon juice, olive oil, and Dijon mustard to make the dressing.
4. In a large mixing bowl, combine the mixed greens, avocado slices, and sunflower seeds. Drizzle with the dressing and toss gently to coat.
5. Divide the salad between two plates and top with the sliced roasted chicken. Serve immediately.

Chef's Tip:

- For added flavor, season the chicken with paprika or garlic powder before roasting.

Thyroid Health Note: This salad is a powerhouse of nutrients. Chicken provides lean protein for sustained energy, while avocado delivers healthy fats to support hormone production. Sunflower seeds are rich in selenium, an essential mineral for thyroid health, making this meal both delicious and functional.

Vegetarian Buddha Bowl with Spiced Chickpeas and Hummus

This colorful and nutrient-packed Buddha bowl is a vegetarian delight, featuring spiced chickpeas, creamy hummus, and a variety of fresh vegetables. It's a perfect balance of protein, fiber, and healthy fats to support energy and thyroid health.

Serves: 2 | **Prep Time**: 10 minutes | **Cook Time**: 15 minutes | **Equipment Needed**: Baking sheet, mixing bowl, knife, cutting board | **Nutritional Information**: 400 calories (per serving), 15g protein, 35g carbohydrates, 18g fat

Ingredients:

- 1 cup (200g) cooked chickpeas, drained and rinsed
- 1 tablespoon (15ml) olive oil
- 1 teaspoon (2g) ground cumin
- 1/2 teaspoon (1g) smoked paprika
- 1/4 teaspoon (1g) salt
- 2 cups (60g) mixed greens (e.g., spinach, arugula, kale)
- 1/2 cup (100g) cooked quinoa
- 1/2 cup (120g) cherry tomatoes, halved
- 1/2 cucumber (about 100g), sliced
- 1/4 avocado (about 50g), sliced
- 1/4 cup (60g) hummus
- 1 tablespoon (15ml) lemon juice
- 1 teaspoon (5ml) tahini (optional, for drizzling)

Instructions:

1. Preheat your oven to 400°F (200°C). Line a baking sheet with parchment paper.
2. In a mixing bowl, toss the chickpeas with olive oil, cumin, smoked paprika, and salt. Spread them in a single layer on the baking sheet and roast for 15 minutes, or until crispy.
3. Assemble the Buddha bowl: Start with a base of mixed greens and cooked quinoa. Arrange the cherry tomatoes, cucumber, avocado slices, and roasted chickpeas on top.
4. Add a dollop of hummus in the center and drizzle with lemon juice and tahini if desired. Serve immediately.

Chef's Tip:

- For extra crunch, sprinkle sunflower seeds or chopped nuts over the bowl.
- To save time, use store-bought roasted chickpeas or prep them in advance.

Thyroid Health Note: This bowl is a nutrient powerhouse. Chickpeas provide plant-based protein and zinc, while quinoa adds complete amino acids and fiber. Hummus and avocado offer healthy fats to support hormone production and reduce inflammation.

Garlic Butter Shrimp with Zucchini Noodles

Quick, flavorful, and low in carbohydrates, this garlic butter shrimp with zucchini noodles is a perfect dinner option for anyone looking for a light yet satisfying meal. Packed with protein and healthy fats, it supports thyroid health and promotes energy balance.

Serves: 2 | **Prep Time**: 10 minutes | **Cook Time**: 10 minutes | **Equipment Needed**: Spiralizer, skillet, knife, cutting board | **Nutritional Information**: 350 calories (per serving), 28g protein, 10g carbohydrates, 22g fat

Ingredients:

- 12 large shrimp (about 200g), peeled and deveined
- 2 medium zucchinis (about 300g), spiralized
- 2 tablespoons (30g) unsalted butter
- 3 garlic cloves, minced
- 1/4 teaspoon (1g) red pepper flakes (optional)
- 1/2 teaspoon (1g) salt
- 1/4 teaspoon (1g) black pepper
- Juice of 1/2 lemon (about 1 tablespoon or 15ml)
- 1 tablespoon (4g) fresh parsley, chopped (optional, for garnish)

Instructions:

1. Heat 1 tablespoon of butter in a skillet over medium heat. Add the minced garlic and red pepper flakes (if using) and sauté for 1-2 minutes until fragrant.
2. Add the shrimp to the skillet, season with salt and pepper, and cook for 2-3 minutes per side until pink and fully cooked. Remove the shrimp from the skillet and set aside.
3. In the same skillet, add the remaining butter and the zucchini noodles. Cook for 2-3 minutes, tossing gently, until the noodles are tender but not mushy.
4. Return the shrimp to the skillet, squeeze in the lemon juice, and toss everything together to combine.
5. Serve immediately, garnished with fresh parsley if desired.

Chef's Tip:

- To enhance the flavor, add a splash of white wine while cooking the shrimp.
- Use pre-spiralized zucchini to save prep time.

Thyroid Health Note: Shrimp is an excellent source of iodine and selenium, both essential for thyroid hormone production and immune support. Zucchini noodles provide a low carb base rich in antioxidants and fiber, making this dish light, flavorful, and thyroid-friendly.

Herb-Roasted Chicken with Sweet Potatoes

This herb-roasted chicken with sweet potatoes is a comforting and flavorful meal that's easy to prepare. Packed with protein, healthy fats, and complex carbohydrates, it's perfect for supporting energy and thyroid health.

Serves: 4 | **Prep Time**: 15 minutes | **Cook Time**: 40 minutes | **Equipment Needed**: Baking sheet, mixing bowl, knife, cutting board | **Nutritional Information**: 380 calories (per serving), 30g protein, 25g carbohydrates, 18g fat

Ingredients:

- 4 bone-in, skin-on chicken thighs (about 600g)
- 2 medium sweet potatoes (about 300g), peeled and cubed
- 1 tablespoon (15ml) olive oil
- 1 teaspoon (2g) dried rosemary
- 1 teaspoon (2g) dried thyme
- 1/2 teaspoon (1g) garlic powder
- 1/2 teaspoon (1g) paprika
- 1/2 teaspoon (1g) salt
- 1/4 teaspoon (1g) black pepper

Instructions:

1. Preheat your oven to 400°F (200°C). Line a baking sheet with parchment paper.
2. In a mixing bowl, toss the sweet potatoes with 1/2 tablespoon of olive oil, rosemary, thyme, garlic powder, paprika, salt, and pepper. Spread them evenly on the prepared baking sheet.
3. Rub the chicken thighs with the remaining olive oil and season with salt and pepper. Place the chicken on the baking sheet alongside the sweet potatoes.
4. Roast in the oven for 35-40 minutes, or until the chicken reaches an internal temperature of 165°F (74°C) and the sweet potatoes are tender and slightly caramelized.
5. Remove from the oven and let rest for 5 minutes before serving. Pair with a simple side salad or steamed greens for a complete meal.

Chef's Tip:

- For added flavor, squeeze fresh lemon juice over the chicken and sweet potatoes before serving.

Thyroid Health Note: This dish is rich in protein and healthy fats from the chicken, while sweet potatoes provide complex carbohydrates and beta-carotene, essential for immune support and energy. The herbs add anti-inflammatory benefits, making this meal as nutritious as it is delicious.

Lemon-Baked Salmon with Broccoli and Cauliflower

This lemon-baked salmon with broccoli and cauliflower is a quick, healthy, and flavorful dish. High in omega-3 fatty acids and loaded with antioxidants, it's a perfect meal to support thyroid function and overall health.

Serves: 2 | **Prep Time**: 10 minutes | **Cook Time**: 20 minutes | **Equipment Needed**: Baking dish, knife, cutting board, foil or parchment paper | **Nutritional Information**: 350 calories (per serving), 28g protein, 12g carbohydrates, 20g fat

Ingredients:

- 2 salmon fillets (about 300g total)
- 1 small head of broccoli (about 200g), cut into florets
- 1 small head of cauliflower (about 200g), cut into florets
- 2 tablespoons (30ml) olive oil
- Juice and zest of 1 lemon (about 2 tablespoons or 30ml juice)
- 1 teaspoon (2g) garlic powder
- 1/2 teaspoon (1g) salt
- 1/4 teaspoon (1g) black pepper
- Fresh parsley for garnish (optional)

Instructions:

1. Preheat your oven to 375°F (190°C). Line a baking dish with foil or parchment paper.
2. Arrange the broccoli and cauliflower florets in the baking dish. Drizzle with 1 tablespoon of olive oil and season with garlic powder, salt, and pepper. Toss to coat evenly.
3. Place the salmon fillets on top of the vegetables. Drizzle with the remaining olive oil, lemon juice, and sprinkle with lemon zest.
4. Cover the dish with foil and bake for 15 minutes. Remove the foil and bake for an additional 5 minutes, or until the salmon is cooked through and flakes easily with a fork.
5. Garnish with fresh parsley before serving. Pair with quinoa or brown rice for a complete meal.

Chef's Tip:

- For a crispier texture, broil the salmon and vegetables for 2-3 minutes after baking.

Thyroid Health Note:

Salmon is an excellent source of omega-3 fatty acids, which reduce inflammation and support thyroid hormone production. Broccoli and cauliflower provide antioxidants and fiber, while the lemon adds vitamin C to enhance iron absorption and immune support.

Beef Stir-Fry with Asian Vegetables and Ginger Sauce

This quick and flavorful beef stir-fry is a perfect weeknight meal, featuring tender beef, colorful vegetables, and a savory ginger sauce. It's packed with protein and antioxidants to support thyroid health and overall energy.

Serves: 2-3 | **Prep Time**: 15 minutes | **Cook Time**: 10 minutes | **Equipment Needed**: Wok or large skillet, knife, cutting board | **Nutritional Information**: 350 calories (per serving), 28g protein, 15g carbohydrates, 18g fat

Ingredients:

- 300g beef sirloin, thinly sliced
- 1 small red bell pepper (about 100g), thinly sliced
- 1 cup (150g) broccoli florets
- 2 garlic cloves, minced
- 2 tablespoons (30ml) tamari or low-sodium soy sauce
- 1 teaspoon (5ml) honey (optional)
- 1/4 teaspoon (1g) red pepper flakes (optional)
- 2 tablespoons (30ml) coconut oil or olive oil
- 1 medium carrot (about 80g), julienned
- 1/2 cup (100g) snow peas, trimmed
- 1 tablespoon (15g) grated fresh ginger
- 1 tablespoon (15ml) sesame oil
- 1 teaspoon (5ml) rice vinegar
- Sesame seeds and green onions for garnish (optional)

Instructions:

1. Heat 1 tablespoon of coconut oil in a wok or large skillet over medium-high heat. Add the beef and stir-fry for 2-3 minutes until browned. Remove the beef from the pan and set aside.
2. Add the remaining coconut oil to the wok. Stir-fry the bell pepper, carrot, broccoli, and snow peas for 3-4 minutes, until tender-crisp.
3. In a small bowl, whisk together the tamari, sesame oil, honey, rice vinegar, garlic, ginger, and red pepper flakes.
4. Return the beef to the wok and pour the sauce over the stir-fry. Toss to combine and cook for an additional 1-2 minutes, until heated through.
5. Serve immediately, garnished with sesame seeds and green onions if desired. Pair with steamed rice or cauliflower rice for a complete meal.

Chef's Tip:

- For extra flavor, marinate the beef in a mixture of tamari, garlic, and ginger for 30 minutes before cooking.

Thyroid Health Note: This stir-fry is rich in selenium and zinc from the beef, which support thyroid hormone production. The variety of vegetables adds antioxidants and fiber to reduce inflammation and promote digestion, while ginger boosts circulation and immune health.

Spinach and Mushroom-Stuffed Chicken Breast

This elegant yet simple dish features tender chicken breasts stuffed with a savory mixture of spinach, mushrooms, and herbs. It's high in protein and nutrients, making it a perfect choice for a healthy dinner.

Serves: 2 | **Prep Time**: 15 minutes | **Cook Time**: 30 minutes | **Equipment Needed**: Baking dish, skillet, knife, cutting board, toothpicks | **Nutritional Information**: 400 calories (per serving), 35g protein, 8g carbohydrates, 20g fat

Ingredients:

- 2 large chicken breasts (about 300g total), butterflied
- 1 tablespoon (15ml) olive oil
- 1 cup (30g) fresh spinach, chopped
- 1/2 cup (80g) mushrooms, finely chopped
- 2 garlic cloves, minced
- 1/4 teaspoon (1g) salt
- 1/4 teaspoon (1g) black pepper
- 1/4 teaspoon (1g) dried thyme
- 1/4 cup (30g) grated dairy-free cheese (optional)

Instructions:

1. Preheat your oven to 375°F (190°C). Lightly grease a baking dish with olive oil.
2. Heat 1/2 tablespoon of olive oil in a skillet over medium heat. Add the mushrooms, spinach, garlic, thyme, salt, and pepper. Cook for 3-4 minutes, until the vegetables are tender and the spinach is wilted. Remove from heat and let cool slightly.
3. Spread the spinach and mushroom mixture evenly inside each butterflied chicken breast. If using, sprinkle the grated cheese on top of the filling.
4. Fold the chicken breasts closed and secure the edges with toothpicks. Place them in the prepared baking dish.
5. Brush the top of the chicken with the remaining olive oil and bake for 25-30 minutes, or until the internal temperature reaches 165°F (74°C).
6. Remove the chicken from the oven and let rest for 5 minutes before slicing. Serve warm with a side of roasted vegetables or a fresh salad.

Chef's Tip:

- For a crispy topping, sprinkle gluten free breadcrumbs over the stuffed chicken before baking.
- Store leftovers in the fridge for up to 3 days. Reheat in the oven to maintain texture.

Thyroid Health Note: This stuffed chicken breast is high in protein, which is essential for muscle repair and energy. Spinach and mushrooms provide magnesium, selenium, and antioxidants to reduce inflammation and support thyroid function, making this dish both delicious and nutritious.

Sweet Potato and Lentil Shepherd's Pie

This plant-based twist on a classic shepherd's pie is hearty, satisfying, and loaded with nutrients. Lentils and vegetables create a savory filling, topped with creamy mashed sweet potatoes for a comforting meal.

Serves: 4 | **Prep Time**: 20 minutes | **Cook Time**: 40 minutes | **Equipment Needed**: Large skillet, baking dish, potato masher | **Nutritional Information**: 320 calories (per serving), 12g protein, 50g carbohydrates, 8g fat

Ingredients

For the filling:

- 1 tablespoon (15ml) olive oil
- 2 garlic cloves, minced
- 1 celery stalk (about 50g), diced
- 1 cup (240ml) vegetable broth
- 1 teaspoon (2g) dried thyme
- 1/2 teaspoon (1g) salt
- 1 small onion (about 100g), diced
- 1 medium carrot (about 80g), diced
- 1 cup (200g) cooked lentils (green or brown)
- 1 tablespoon (15g) tomato paste
- 1/2 teaspoon (1g) paprika
- 1/4 teaspoon (1g) black pepper

For the topping:

- 2 medium sweet potatoes (about 400g), peeled and cubed
- 2 tablespoons (30ml) unsweetened almond milk
- 1 tablespoon (15ml) olive oil
- 1/4 teaspoon (1g) salt

Instructions

1. Preheat your oven to 375°F (190°C).
2. Heat olive oil in a large skillet over medium heat. Add the onion, garlic, carrot, and celery. Cook for 5-7 minutes until softened.
3. Stir in the lentils, vegetable broth, tomato paste, thyme, paprika, salt, and pepper. Simmer for 10 minutes, or until the mixture thickens slightly.
4. Meanwhile, boil the sweet potatoes in a pot of water for 15 minutes, or until tender. Drain and mash with almond milk, olive oil, and salt.
5. Transfer the lentil mixture to a baking dish. Spread the mashed sweet potatoes on top, smoothing with a spoon. Bake for 20 minutes, or until the topping is lightly golden. Serve warm.

Chef's Tip: Add a sprinkle of smoked paprika on top of the mashed sweet potatoes before baking.

Thyroid Health Note: Sweet potatoes provide complex carbohydrates and beta-carotene, essential for immune health. Lentils are a great source of plant-based protein and iron, supporting energy levels and thyroid function.

Eggplant and Chickpea Stew with Tomatoes and Spices

This hearty stew combines tender eggplant, protein-packed chickpeas, and aromatic spices for a flavorful and nourishing meal. Perfect with a side of gluten-free bread or rice.

Serves: 4 | **Prep Time**: 15 minutes | **Cook Time**: 30 minutes | **Equipment Needed**: Large pot, wooden spoon | **Nutritional Information**: 280 calories (per serving), 8g protein, 35g carbohydrates, 10g fat

Ingredients:

- 1 tablespoon (15ml) olive oil
- 1 medium onion (about 100g), diced
- 2 garlic cloves, minced
- 1 medium eggplant (about 300g), diced
- 1 red bell pepper (about 100g), diced
- 1 can (400g) diced tomatoes
- 1 cup (200g) cooked chickpeas
- 1 teaspoon (2g) ground cumin
- 1/2 teaspoon (1g) smoked paprika
- 1/2 teaspoon (1g) salt
- 1/4 teaspoon (1g) black pepper
- 1/4 cup (15g) fresh parsley, chopped (optional, for garnish)

Instructions:

1. Heat olive oil in a large pot over medium heat. Add the onion and garlic, cooking for 3-4 minutes until softened.
2. Stir in the eggplant and red bell pepper. Cook for 8-10 minutes until the vegetables begin to soften.
3. Add the diced tomatoes, chickpeas, cumin, smoked paprika, salt, and pepper. Stir to combine.
4. Simmer for 15 minutes, stirring occasionally, until the eggplant is tender and the flavors meld together.
5. Serve hot, garnished with fresh parsley if desired.

Chef's Tip:

- For added depth of flavor, roast the eggplant before adding it to the stew.
- Leftovers taste even better the next day as the flavors deepen.

Thyroid Health Note:

Eggplant and chickpeas are rich in fiber and antioxidants, supporting digestion and reducing inflammation. The spices in this stew, such as cumin and paprika, promote circulation and immune health.

Mushroom and Spinach Risotto (Dairy-Free)

This creamy, dairy-free risotto is packed with earthy mushrooms and fresh spinach for a comforting, nutrient-rich dish that's naturally gluten-free.

Serves: 4 | **Prep Time**: 10 minutes | **Cook Time**: 30 minutes | **Equipment Needed**: Large skillet, wooden spoon | **Nutritional Information**: 350 calories (per serving), 8g protein, 45g carbohydrates, 12g fat

Ingredients:

- 1 tablespoon (15ml) olive oil
- 1 small onion (about 100g), finely diced
- 2 garlic cloves, minced
- 1 cup (200g) arborio rice
- 1/2 cup (120ml) dry white wine (optional)
- 3 cups (720ml) vegetable broth, warmed
- 1 cup (100g) mushrooms, sliced
- 2 cups (60g) fresh spinach
- 1/4 teaspoon (1g) salt
- 1/4 teaspoon (1g) black pepper

Instructions:

1. Heat olive oil in a large skillet over medium heat. Add the onion and garlic, cooking for 3-4 minutes until softened.
2. Stir in the arborio rice and cook for 1-2 minutes until lightly toasted. Add the white wine, stirring until absorbed.
3. Gradually add the warm vegetable broth, one ladle at a time, stirring frequently until absorbed before adding more.
4. After 15 minutes, stir in the mushrooms and cook for an additional 5 minutes. Add the spinach, salt, and pepper, cooking until the spinach wilts.
5. Serve hot, garnished with fresh herbs if desired.

Chef's Tip:

- Add a squeeze of lemon juice at the end of cooking for a bright finish.
- Use nutritional yeast for a cheesy flavor without dairy.

Thyroid Health Note: Spinach provides magnesium and iron, essential for thyroid function and energy. Mushrooms are rich in selenium and antioxidants, making this risotto both comforting and supportive of overall health.

Lentil and Sweet Potato Patties

These flavorful patties are crispy on the outside and tender on the inside. Packed with protein and fiber, they're perfect as a main dish or a snack.

Serves: 4 | **Prep Time**: 15 minutes | **Cook Time**: 15 minutes | **Equipment Needed**: Mixing bowl, skillet | **Nutritional Information**: 250 calories (per serving), 10g protein, 40g carbohydrates, 6g fat

Ingredients:

- 1 cup (200g) cooked lentils
- 1 cup (200g) mashed sweet potatoes
- 1/4 cup (30g) gluten-free breadcrumbs
- 1/4 teaspoon (1g) ground cumin
- 1/4 teaspoon (1g) smoked paprika
- 1/2 teaspoon (1g) salt
- 1/4 teaspoon (1g) black pepper
- 2 tablespoons (30ml) olive oil (for frying)

Instructions:

1. In a mixing bowl, combine the lentils, mashed sweet potatoes, breadcrumbs, cumin, smoked paprika, salt, and pepper. Mix until well combined.
2. Form the mixture into 8 small patties.
3. Heat olive oil in a skillet over medium heat. Cook the patties for 3-4 minutes per side, or until golden brown and crispy.
4. Serve warm with a side salad or a dipping sauce of choice.

Chef's Tip:

- Serve these patties with a dollop of dairy-free yogurt or a drizzle of tahini for added flavor.
- Freeze uncooked patties for a quick meal prep option.

Thyroid Health Note: Lentils are rich in plant-based protein and fiber, while sweet potatoes provide beta-carotene and complex carbohydrates for sustained energy. This dish is a thyroid-friendly, nutrient-dense choice.

Zucchini Lasagna with Turkey and Spinach

This light and flavorful zucchini lasagna is a delicious low-carb alternative to the classic dish. Layers of zucchini, turkey, and spinach make it protein-packed and satisfying.

Serves: 4 | **Prep Time**: 20 minutes | **Cook Time**: 40 minutes | **Equipment Needed**: Baking dish, mandoline or sharp knife, skillet | **Nutritional Information**: 300 calories (per serving), 25g protein, 12g carbohydrates, 18g fat

Ingredients:

- 3 medium zucchinis (about 600g), sliced lengthwise into thin strips
- 1 tablespoon (15ml) olive oil
- 1 small onion (about 100g), diced
- 2 garlic cloves, minced
- 1 pound (450g) ground turkey
- 1 teaspoon (2g) dried oregano
- 1/2 teaspoon (1g) paprika
- 1/2 teaspoon (1g) salt
- 1/4 teaspoon (1g) black pepper
- 2 cups (480g) marinara sauce (sugar-free)
- 2 cups (60g) fresh spinach leaves
- 1/2 cup (50g) shredded dairy-free cheese (optional)

Instructions:

1. Preheat your oven to 375°F (190°C).
2. Heat olive oil in a skillet over medium heat. Add the onion and garlic, cooking for 3-4 minutes until softened. Add the ground turkey, oregano, paprika, salt, and pepper. Cook for 7-8 minutes, breaking up the turkey, until fully cooked.
3. Spread a thin layer of marinara sauce on the bottom of a baking dish. Layer zucchini strips, followed by turkey, spinach, and more marinara. Repeat layers, ending with zucchini and marinara on top. Sprinkle cheese, if using.
4. Cover with foil and bake for 25 minutes. Remove the foil and bake for an additional 15 minutes, until bubbly and golden.
5. Let rest for 5 minutes before slicing and serving.

Chef's Tip:

- Salt the zucchini slices and let them sit for 10 minutes to release excess moisture. Pat dry before layering.
- Add fresh basil or parsley for extra flavor.

Thyroid Health Note: Zucchini is low in carbs and high in antioxidants, while turkey provides lean protein to support muscle repair. Spinach offers magnesium and iron, essential for thyroid function.

Cauliflower Steak with Chimichurri Sauce

These roasted cauliflower steaks are served with a zesty chimichurri sauce for a flavorful and nutrient-packed dish. Perfect as a main or side.

Serves: 2 | **Prep Time**: 10 minutes | **Cook Time**: 30 minutes | **Equipment Needed**: Baking sheet, blender or food processor | **Nutritional Information**: 200 calories (per serving), 4g protein, 14g carbohydrates, 14g fat

Ingredients

For the cauliflower:

- 1 large head of cauliflower, sliced into 1-inch (2.5cm) steaks
- 2 tablespoons (30ml) olive oil
- 1/2 teaspoon (1g) smoked paprika
- 1/2 teaspoon (1g) salt
- 1/4 teaspoon (1g) black pepper

For the chimichurri sauce:

- 1/2 cup (15g) fresh parsley
- 1/4 cup (10g) fresh cilantro
- 1 garlic clove, minced
- 2 tablespoons (30ml) olive oil
- 1 tablespoon (15ml) red wine vinegar
- 1/4 teaspoon (1g) salt
- 1/4 teaspoon (1g) red pepper flakes (optional)

Instructions

1. Preheat your oven to 400°F (200°C). Line a baking sheet with parchment paper.
2. Brush the cauliflower steaks with olive oil and sprinkle with smoked paprika, salt, and pepper. Arrange on the baking sheet and roast for 25-30 minutes, flipping halfway, until golden and tender.
3. Meanwhile, prepare the chimichurri sauce by blending all the ingredients in a food processor until smooth.
4. Serve the cauliflower steaks drizzled with chimichurri sauce.

Chef's Tip

- For extra crispiness, broil the cauliflower for 2-3 minutes after roasting.
- Save the smaller cauliflower florets and roast them alongside the steaks.

Thyroid Health Note: Cauliflower is rich in antioxidants and fiber, supporting digestion and reducing inflammation. Chimichurri sauce adds healthy fats and fresh herbs to enhance thyroid function.

Shrimp Scampi with Spaghetti Squash

This light and flavorful shrimp scampi is served over spaghetti squash, making it a perfect low-carb dinner option that doesn't skimp on taste.

Serves: 2 | **Prep Time**: 10 minutes | **Cook Time**: 30 minutes | **Equipment Needed**: Baking sheet, skillet, fork | **Nutritional Information**: 320 calories (per serving), 25g protein, 10g carbohydrates, 18g fat

Ingredients

- 1 medium spaghetti squash (about 600g)
- 1 tablespoon (15ml) olive oil
- 2 garlic cloves, minced
- 12 large shrimp (about 200g), peeled and deveined
- 1/4 teaspoon (1g) red pepper flakes (optional)
- Juice of 1/2 lemon (about 1 tablespoon or 15ml)
- 1/4 cup (15g) fresh parsley, chopped
- 1/2 teaspoon (1g) salt
- 1/4 teaspoon (1g) black pepper

Instructions

1. Preheat your oven to 400°F (200°C). Cut the spaghetti squash in half lengthwise, scoop out the seeds, and place cut-side down on a baking sheet. Roast for 25-30 minutes, or until tender.
2. Meanwhile, heat olive oil in a skillet over medium heat. Add garlic and red pepper flakes (if using), cooking for 1 minute until fragrant.
3. Add the shrimp, salt, and pepper. Cook for 2-3 minutes per side, until pink and opaque. Stir in lemon juice and parsley.
4. Use a fork to scrape the spaghetti squash into strands. Serve topped with shrimp scampi.

Chef's Tip

- Sprinkle grated dairy-free cheese on top for added flavor.
- Prepare the spaghetti squash in advance to save time.

Thyroid Health Note: Shrimp is rich in iodine and selenium, essential for thyroid hormone production. Spaghetti squash provides a low-carb base and is high in antioxidants.

Salmon Patties with Dill Yogurt Sauce

These crispy salmon patties are paired with a refreshing dill yogurt sauce for a flavorful and protein-packed meal.

Serves: 4 | **Prep Time**: 15 minutes | **Cook Time**: 15 minutes | **Equipment Needed**: Mixing bowl, skillet | **Nutritional Information**: 280 calories (per serving), 20g protein, 8g carbohydrates, 18g fat

Ingredients

For the patties:

- 1 can (200g) salmon, drained and flaked
- 1/2 cup (50g) gluten-free breadcrumbs
- 1 egg, beaten
- 1 tablespoon (15ml) Dijon mustard
- 1 tablespoon (15g) chopped fresh dill
- 1/2 teaspoon (1g) garlic powder
- 1/4 teaspoon (1g) salt
- 1/4 teaspoon (1g) black pepper
- 2 tablespoons (30ml) olive oil (for frying)

For the sauce:

- 1/2 cup (120g) dairy-free yogurt
- 1 tablespoon (15ml) lemon juice
- 1 tablespoon (15g) chopped fresh dill

Instructions

1. In a mixing bowl, combine all patty ingredients except the olive oil. Form the mixture into 8 small patties.
2. Heat olive oil in a skillet over medium heat. Fry the patties for 3-4 minutes per side, or until golden and crispy.
3. In a small bowl, whisk together the yogurt, lemon juice, and dill for the sauce.
4. Serve the salmon patties warm with the dill yogurt sauce.

Chef's Tip

- Add a pinch of smoked paprika to the patties for extra depth of flavor.
- Serve with a side salad or roasted vegetables for a complete meal.

Thyroid Health Note: Salmon is a powerhouse of omega-3s and selenium, both crucial for thyroid health. The dill yogurt sauce adds freshness and supports digestion.

Thai Green Curry with Vegetables and Coconut Milk

This aromatic Thai green curry is packed with fresh vegetables and creamy coconut milk, making it a flavorful and satisfying meal. Perfect for a quick and nutritious dinner.

Serves: 4 | **Prep Time**: 15 minutes | **Cook Time**: 20 minutes | **Equipment Needed**: Large skillet, wooden spoon | **Nutritional Information**: 320 calories (per serving), 6g protein, 22g carbohydrates, 24g fat

Ingredients

- 1 tablespoon (15ml) coconut oil
- 1 small onion (about 100g), sliced
- 2 garlic cloves, minced
- 1 tablespoon (15g) green curry paste
- 1 can (400ml) full-fat coconut milk
- 1 cup (240ml) vegetable broth
- 1 medium zucchini (about 200g), sliced
- 1 red bell pepper (about 100g), sliced
- 1 cup (150g) green beans, trimmed
- 1/4 cup (10g) fresh basil leaves
- Juice of 1/2 lime (about 1 tablespoon or 15ml)
- 1/2 teaspoon (1g) salt
- Cooked jasmine rice (optional, for serving)

Instructions

1. Heat coconut oil in a large skillet over medium heat. Add the onion and garlic, cooking for 2-3 minutes until fragrant.
2. Stir in the green curry paste and cook for 1 minute to release its aroma.
3. Add the coconut milk, vegetable broth, zucchini, bell pepper, and green beans. Bring to a simmer and cook for 10-12 minutes, or until the vegetables are tender.
4. Stir in the basil leaves, lime juice, and salt. Adjust seasoning as needed.
5. Serve hot, with cooked jasmine rice if desired.

Chef's Tip

- For added protein, stir in cooked tofu or shredded chicken during the last 5 minutes of cooking.
- Garnish with extra basil leaves or a sprinkle of chili flakes for a spicy kick.

Thyroid Health Note: Coconut milk provides healthy fats that support hormone production, while the vegetables add antioxidants and fiber. The green curry paste enhances circulation and supports digestion.

Moroccan Chickpea Tagine with Apricots and Almonds

This sweet and savory Moroccan tagine combines chickpeas, apricots, and almonds with warm spices for a dish bursting with flavor. Serve with gluten-free couscous or rice for a complete meal.

Serves: 4 | **Prep Time**: 10 minutes | **Cook Time**: 30 minutes | **Equipment Needed**: Large pot, wooden spoon | **Nutritional Information**: 340 calories (per serving), 10g protein, 50g carbohydrates, 10g fat

Ingredients

- 1 tablespoon (15ml) olive oil
- 1 small onion (about 100g), diced
- 2 garlic cloves, minced
- 1 teaspoon (2g) ground cumin
- 1 teaspoon (2g) ground cinnamon
- 1/2 teaspoon (1g) ground turmeric
- 1 can (400g) diced tomatoes
- 1 cup (200g) cooked chickpeas
- 1/2 cup (75g) dried apricots, chopped
- 1/4 cup (30g) slivered almonds
- 1 cup (240ml) vegetable broth
- 1/2 teaspoon (1g) salt
- 1/4 teaspoon (1g) black pepper
- Fresh cilantro (optional, for garnish)

Instructions

1. Heat olive oil in a large pot over medium heat. Add the onion and garlic, cooking for 3-4 minutes until softened.
2. Stir in the cumin, cinnamon, and turmeric. Cook for 1 minute until fragrant.
3. Add the diced tomatoes, chickpeas, apricots, almonds, vegetable broth, salt, and pepper. Stir to combine.
4. Simmer for 20-25 minutes, stirring occasionally, until the sauce thickens and the flavors meld.
5. Serve hot, garnished with fresh cilantro if desired.

Chef's Tip

- For added depth of flavor, toast the almonds in a dry skillet before adding them to the tagine.
- Pair with a side of gluten-free couscous or quinoa for a hearty meal.

Thyroid Health Note: Chickpeas provide plant-based protein and fiber, while apricots add natural sweetness and antioxidants. The spices support circulation and reduce inflammation, making this dish both flavorful and nourishing.

Indian-Spiced Lentil Dhal with Coconut Rice

This creamy dhal is made with red lentils and a blend of warming spices, served alongside fragrant coconut rice for a comforting and nutrient-rich meal.

Serves: 4 | **Prep Time**: 10 minutes | **Cook Time**: 30 minutes | **Equipment Needed**: Large pot, wooden spoon, medium saucepan | **Nutritional Information**: 360 calories (per serving), 12g protein, 50g carbohydrates, 12g fat

Ingredients

For the dhal:

- 1 tablespoon (15ml) coconut oil
- 2 garlic cloves, minced
- 1 teaspoon (2g) ground cumin
- 1/2 teaspoon (1g) ground turmeric
- 3 cups (720ml) vegetable broth
- 1/4 teaspoon (1g) chili powder (optional)
- 1 small onion (about 100g), diced
- 1 tablespoon (15g) grated fresh ginger
- 1 teaspoon (2g) ground coriander
- 1 cup (200g) red lentils, rinsed
- 1/2 teaspoon (1g) salt

For the coconut rice:

- 1 cup (200g) basmati rice
- 1 1/2 cups (360ml) water
- 1/2 cup (120ml) coconut milk
- 1/4 teaspoon (1g) salt

Instructions

1. Heat coconut oil in a large pot over medium heat. Add the onion, garlic, and ginger, cooking for 3-4 minutes until fragrant.
2. Stir in the cumin, coriander, and turmeric. Cook for 1 minute to release their aroma.
3. Add the lentils, vegetable broth, salt, and chili powder (if using). Simmer for 20-25 minutes, stirring occasionally, until the lentils are soft and the dhal is creamy.
4. Meanwhile, combine the rice, water, coconut milk, and salt in a medium saucepan. Bring to a boil, then reduce heat to low, cover, and cook for 15 minutes, or until the liquid is absorbed.
5. Serve the dhal over the coconut rice, garnished with fresh cilantro if desired.

Chef's Tip

- Add a squeeze of lime juice to the dhal for a bright, tangy finish.
- Leftovers can be stored in the fridge for up to 3 days and reheated gently on the stovetop.

Thyroid Health Note: Lentils provide plant-based protein and iron, while the coconut milk in the rice offers healthy fats that support thyroid function. The spices promote circulation and digestive health.

Spanish-Style Garlic Shrimp (Gambas al Ajillo)

These Spanish-style garlic shrimp are simple yet bursting with flavor, thanks to fresh garlic, olive oil, and a touch of paprika. Serve as an appetizer or a light meal.

Serves: 2 | **Prep Time**: 5 minutes | **Cook Time**: 10 minutes | **Equipment Needed**: Skillet, wooden spoon | **Nutritional Information**: 280 calories (per serving), 20g protein, 4g carbohydrates, 22g fat

Ingredients

- 2 tablespoons (30ml) olive oil
- 4 garlic cloves, thinly sliced
- 12 large shrimp (about 200g), peeled and deveined
- 1/4 teaspoon (1g) smoked paprika
- 1/4 teaspoon (1g) red pepper flakes (optional)
- Juice of 1/2 lemon (about 1 tablespoon or 15ml)
- 1 tablespoon (15g) chopped fresh parsley
- 1/4 teaspoon (1g) salt
- Gluten-free bread or steamed vegetables (optional, for serving)

Instructions

1. Heat olive oil in a skillet over medium heat. Add the garlic and cook for 1-2 minutes until fragrant and golden.
2. Stir in the shrimp, smoked paprika, red pepper flakes (if using), and salt. Cook for 2-3 minutes per side, or until the shrimp are pink and opaque.
3. Remove from heat and stir in the lemon juice and parsley.
4. Serve immediately with gluten-free bread or steamed vegetables.

Chef's Tip

- For an authentic touch, serve the shrimp in the skillet they were cooked in.
- Add a splash of white wine to the pan for extra depth of flavor.

Thyroid Health Note: Shrimp is an excellent source of iodine and selenium, essential for thyroid hormone production. The olive oil and garlic provide anti-inflammatory benefits, making

Snacks and Sides

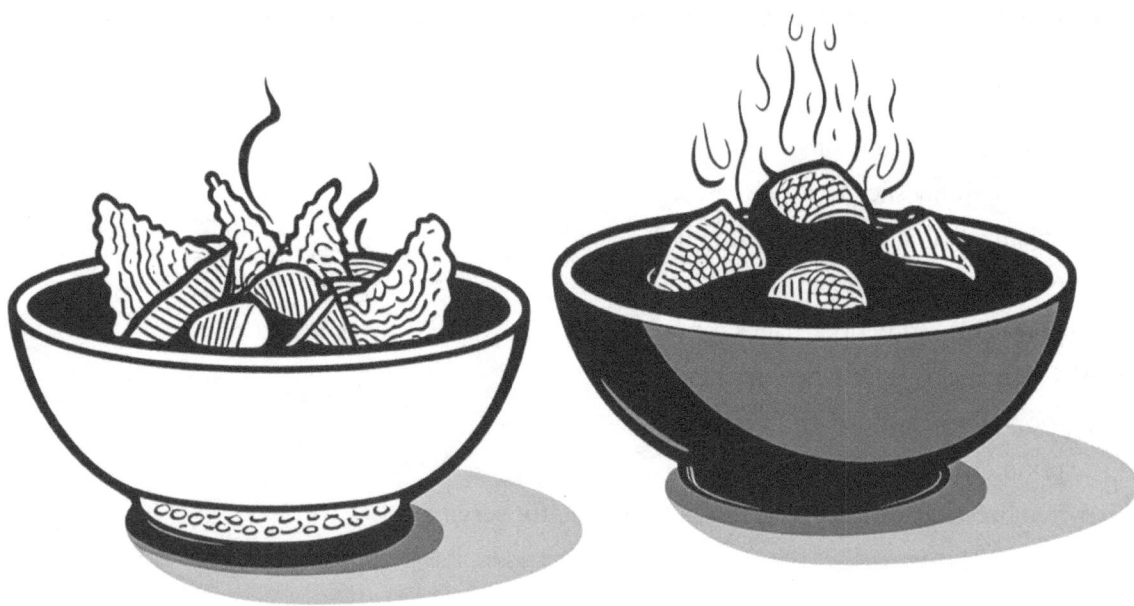

I'm so excited to share these snack and side recipes with you! Making your own snacks and sauces isn't just rewarding—it's a game-changer for your health. Unlike store-bought options that can be loaded with hidden sugars, unhealthy fats, and preservatives, these recipes are fresh, flavorful, and crafted to support your thyroid and overall well-being. Whether you're craving a quick bite or the perfect complement to your meal, these homemade creations will elevate your eating experience while giving you the peace of mind of knowing exactly what's in every bite.

Energy Bites with Chia Seeds, Coconut, and Dates

These no-bake energy bites are a delicious and convenient snack, perfect for a quick energy boost. Packed with fiber, healthy fats, and natural sweetness, they're ideal for busy days and thyroid health support.

Serves: 12 bites | **Prep Time**: 15 minutes | **Equipment Needed**: Food processor, mixing bowl | **Nutritional Information**: 100 calories (per bite), 2g protein, 12g carbohydrates, 5g fat

Ingredients:

- 1 cup (150g) pitted Medjool dates
- 1/2 cup (50g) rolled oats (certified gluten-free)
- 1/4 cup (20g) shredded unsweetened coconut
- 1 tablespoon (10g) chia seeds
- 2 tablespoons (30ml) almond butter
- 1 tablespoon (15ml) maple syrup or honey
- 1/2 teaspoon (1g) ground cinnamon
- A pinch of salt

Instructions:

1. Add the dates to a food processor and pulse until they form a sticky paste.
2. Add the oats, shredded coconut, chia seeds, almond butter, maple syrup, cinnamon, and salt. Process until the mixture comes together and forms a sticky dough.
3. Scoop out 1 tablespoon of the mixture at a time and roll into small balls.
4. Place the energy bites on a plate or baking sheet and refrigerate for at least 30 minutes to firm up.
5. Store in an airtight container in the fridge for up to 1 week or freeze for up to 1 month.

Chef's Tip:

- For extra texture, roll the energy bites in shredded coconut or chia seeds before chilling.
- Add a tablespoon of cocoa powder for a chocolate-flavored variation.

Thyroid Health Note:

These energy bites are rich in omega-3s from chia seeds and healthy fats from almond butter, which support hormonal balance and reduce inflammation. Dates provide natural sweetness and a quick source of energy, making them a great snack for managing fatigue.

Crispy Kale Chips with Olive Oil and Smoked Paprika

Light and crunchy, these crispy kale chips are a healthy alternative to traditional snacks. With just a few ingredients, they're easy to make and packed with antioxidants and fiber to support thyroid health.

Serves: 2 | **Prep Time**: 5 minutes | **Cook Time**: 15 minutes | **Equipment Needed**: Baking sheet, parchment paper, mixing bowl | **Nutritional Information**: 80 calories (per serving), 2g protein, 5g carbohydrates, 6g fat

Ingredients:

- 1 large bunch (200g) kale, stems removed, leaves torn into bite-sized pieces
- 1 tablespoon (15ml) olive oil
- 1/2 teaspoon (1g) smoked paprika
- 1/4 teaspoon (1g) salt
- 1/4 teaspoon (1g) garlic powder (optional)

Instructions:

1. Preheat your oven to 300°F (150°C). Line a baking sheet with parchment paper.
2. In a mixing bowl, toss the kale leaves with olive oil, smoked paprika, salt, and garlic powder (if using) until evenly coated.
3. Spread the kale in a single layer on the prepared baking sheet. Avoid overlapping for even crisping.
4. Bake for 12-15 minutes, checking frequently, until the kale is crispy but not browned.
5. Remove from the oven and let cool for a few minutes before serving.

Chef's Tip:

- For a spicy kick, add a pinch of cayenne pepper to the seasoning.
- Store leftover kale chips in an airtight container for up to 3 days to maintain crispness.

Thyroid Health Note:

Kale is rich in vitamins A, C, and K, as well as antioxidants that reduce oxidative stress. When cooked properly, kale is safe and beneficial for thyroid health, especially when paired with healthy fats like olive oil to enhance nutrient absorption.

Homemade Protein Bars with No Refined Sugar

These homemade protein bars are the perfect snack for busy days. Packed with natural sweetness, healthy fats, and protein, they're ideal for sustained energy without any refined sugar. Make a batch ahead of time for a convenient, thyroid-friendly snack.

Serves: 8 bars | **Prep Time**: 15 minutes | **Chill Time**: 1 hour | **Equipment Needed**: Mixing bowl, food processor, 8x8-inch baking dish, parchment paper | **Nutritional Information**: 200 calories (per bar), 8g protein, 15g carbohydrates, 12g fat

Ingredients:

- 1 cup (150g) pitted Medjool dates
- 1/2 cup (50g) rolled oats (certified gluten-free)
- 1/2 cup (50g) almond flour
- 1/4 cup (60ml) almond butter
- 2 tablespoons (30ml) maple syrup or honey
- 1 scoop (30g) unflavored or vanilla protein powder
- 1/4 teaspoon (1g) salt
- 1/4 teaspoon (1g) ground cinnamon
- 2 tablespoons (30g) dark chocolate chips (optional, for topping)

Instructions:

1. Line an 8x8-inch baking dish with parchment paper.
2. Add the dates to a food processor and pulse until they form a sticky paste.
3. In a mixing bowl, combine the date paste, rolled oats, almond flour, almond butter, maple syrup, protein powder, salt, and cinnamon. Mix until well combined. If the mixture feels too dry, add 1-2 teaspoons of water.
4. Press the mixture firmly into the prepared baking dish, smoothing it out with a spatula.
5. If using, sprinkle the chocolate chips on top and press them lightly into the mixture.
6. Refrigerate for at least 1 hour, or until firm.
7. Remove from the fridge, lift out the parchment paper, and slice into 8 bars. Store in an airtight container in the fridge for up to 1 week or freeze for up to 1 month.

Chef's Tip:

- Add a tablespoon of chia seeds or hemp seeds for an extra nutritional boost.

Thyroid Health Note: These protein bars are made with natural ingredients that support thyroid health. Almond flour and almond butter provide healthy fats and vitamin E, while protein powder helps with muscle repair and energy. The natural sweetness from dates and honey keeps blood sugar stable, making this a balanced and satisfying snack.

Beet and Tahini Hummus

This vibrant beet and tahini hummus is as nutritious as it is beautiful. Packed with antioxidants, fiber, and healthy fats, it's a perfect dip or spread for supporting thyroid health and adding a pop of color to your table.

Serves: 4 | **Prep Time**: 10 minutes | **Equipment Needed**: Food processor, knife, cutting board | **Nutritional Information**: 150 calories (per serving), 4g protein, 12g carbohydrates, 8g fat

Ingredients:

- 1 medium beet (about 150g), cooked and peeled
- 1 cup (150g) cooked chickpeas, drained and rinsed
- 2 tablespoons (30ml) tahini
- Juice of 1 lemon (about 2 tablespoons or 30ml)
- 1 garlic clove, minced
- 2 tablespoons (30ml) olive oil
- 1/2 teaspoon (1g) salt
- 1/4 teaspoon (1g) ground cumin
- 2-3 tablespoons (30-45ml) water (as needed for consistency)

Instructions:

1. If the beet is not already cooked, boil it in water for 30-40 minutes or roast at 400°F/200°C for 45-60 minutes until fork-tender, then peel. Add the cooked beet, chickpeas, tahini, lemon juice, garlic, olive oil, salt, and cumin to a food processor.
2. Blend until smooth, stopping to scrape down the sides as needed. Add water 1 tablespoon at a time until the hummus reaches your desired consistency.
3. Taste and adjust seasoning as needed. Serve immediately or refrigerate for up to 5 days.

Chef's Tip:

- For extra flavor, garnish with a drizzle of olive oil and a sprinkle of sesame seeds or chopped parsley.
- Use this hummus as a dip for fresh veggies, a spread for sandwiches, or a topping for grain bowls.

Thyroid Health Note:

Beets are rich in antioxidants and nitrates, which support circulation and reduce inflammation. Tahini provides healthy fats and calcium, while chickpeas add plant-based protein and fiber, making this hummus both delicious and nutritious.

Avocado Lime Dip

This creamy avocado lime dip is a versatile and flavorful option for snacking or adding a zesty twist to your meals. Loaded with healthy fats and vitamin C, it's both satisfying and supportive of thyroid function.

Serves: 4 | **Prep Time**: 5 minutes | **Equipment Needed**: Blender or food processor, knife, cutting board | **Nutritional Information**: 160 calories (per serving), 2g protein, 8g carbohydrates, 14g fat

Ingredients:

- 2 ripe avocados (about 300g)
- Juice and zest of 1 lime (about 2 tablespoons or 30ml juice)
- 1 garlic clove, minced
- 2 tablespoons (30ml) olive oil
- 1/4 teaspoon (1g) salt
- 1/4 teaspoon (1g) ground cumin
- 1 tablespoon (15ml) water (as needed for consistency)

Instructions:

1. Add the avocados, lime juice, lime zest, garlic, olive oil, salt, and cumin to a blender or food processor.
2. Blend until smooth, adding water 1 tablespoon at a time to adjust the consistency if needed.
3. Taste and adjust seasoning as desired. Serve immediately or refrigerate for up to 3 days.

Chef's Tip:

- Add a pinch of chili powder for a spicy kick or a handful of fresh cilantro for added freshness.
- Use this dip as a topping for tacos, a spread for wraps, or a dip for vegetable sticks.

Thyroid Health Note:

Avocados are a great source of monounsaturated fats, which support hormone production and reduce inflammation. Lime juice adds vitamin C, enhancing immune function and promoting overall wellness.

Spinach and Walnut Pesto (Dairy-Free)

This dairy-free spinach and walnut pesto is a fresh and flavorful sauce perfect for pasta, salads, or roasted vegetables. Packed with antioxidants, healthy fats, and plant-based nutrients, it's a delicious way to support thyroid health.

Serves: 4 | **Prep Time**: 10 minutes | **Equipment Needed**: Blender or food processor, knife, cutting board | **Nutritional Information**: 120 calories (per serving), 3g protein, 2g carbohydrates, 11g fat

Ingredients:

- 2 cups (60g) fresh spinach leaves
- 1/2 cup (50g) walnuts
- 1/4 cup (60ml) olive oil
- 1 garlic clove, minced
- Juice of 1/2 lemon (about 1 tablespoon or 15ml)
- 1/4 teaspoon (1g) salt
- 2 tablespoons (30ml) water (as needed for consistency)

Instructions:

1. Add the spinach, walnuts, olive oil, garlic, lemon juice, and salt to a blender or food processor.
2. Blend until smooth, stopping to scrape down the sides as needed. Add water 1 tablespoon at a time to achieve your desired consistency.
3. Taste and adjust seasoning as necessary. Serve immediately or store in an airtight container in the fridge for up to 5 days.

Chef's Tip:

- For added flavor, mix in a pinch of red pepper flakes or nutritional yeast.
- Use this pesto as a sauce for gluten-free pasta, a spread for sandwiches, or a dip for roasted vegetables.

Thyroid Health Note:

Spinach and walnuts provide antioxidants, magnesium, and healthy fats that support thyroid function and reduce inflammation. Olive oil enhances nutrient absorption, making this pesto both nutritious and versatile.

Roasted Brussels Sprouts with Honey and Balsamic Vinegar

These roasted Brussels sprouts are caramelized to perfection, with a sweet and tangy glaze of honey and balsamic vinegar. They make a delightful side dish that's both flavorful and nutrient-packed.

Serves: 4 | **Prep Time**: 10 minutes | **Cook Time**: 25 minutes | **Equipment Needed**: Baking sheet, mixing bowl, knife, cutting board | **Nutritional Information**: 120 calories (per serving), 3g protein, 15g carbohydrates, 6g fat

Ingredients:

- 1 pound (450g) Brussels sprouts, trimmed and halved
- 2 tablespoons (30ml) olive oil
- 1 tablespoon (15ml) balsamic vinegar
- 1 teaspoon (5ml) honey
- 1/4 teaspoon (1g) salt
- 1/4 teaspoon (1g) black pepper

Instructions:

1. Preheat your oven to 400°F (200°C). Line a baking sheet with parchment paper.
2. In a mixing bowl, toss the Brussels sprouts with olive oil, balsamic vinegar, honey, salt, and pepper until well coated.
3. Spread the Brussels sprouts in a single layer on the prepared baking sheet.
4. Roast for 20-25 minutes, flipping halfway through, until golden brown and crispy on the edges.
5. Serve immediately as a side dish or snack.

Chef's Tip:

- For extra flavor, sprinkle with grated Parmesan or chopped walnuts before serving.
- Add a pinch of red pepper flakes for a spicy kick.

Thyroid Health Note:

Brussels sprouts are a great source of antioxidants and fiber, supporting digestion and reducing oxidative stress. The olive oil enhances nutrient absorption, while the balsamic glaze adds a touch of sweetness without refined sugars.

Grilled Zucchini with Garlic and Thyme

This simple and flavorful side dish features tender grilled zucchini infused with garlic and thyme. It's quick to prepare and complements a variety of main courses.

Serves: 4 | **Prep Time**: 5 minutes | **Cook Time**: 10 minutes | **Equipment Needed**: Grill pan or outdoor grill, mixing bowl, knife, cutting board | **Nutritional Information**: 80 calories (per serving), 2g protein, 4g carbohydrates, 6g fat

Ingredients:

- 4 medium zucchinis (about 600g), sliced lengthwise
- 2 tablespoons (30ml) olive oil
- 2 garlic cloves, minced
- 1 teaspoon (2g) dried thyme
- 1/4 teaspoon (1g) salt
- 1/4 teaspoon (1g) black pepper

Instructions:

1. Preheat your grill or grill pan to medium-high heat.
2. In a mixing bowl, toss the zucchini slices with olive oil, garlic, thyme, salt, and pepper.
3. Place the zucchini on the grill and cook for 3-4 minutes per side, until tender and grill marks appear.
4. Serve warm as a side dish or appetizer.

Chef's Tip:

- For added flavor, drizzle the grilled zucchini with a squeeze of fresh lemon juice before serving.
- Pair with grilled chicken or fish for a complete meal.

Thyroid Health Note:

Zucchini is low in calories and rich in antioxidants, while olive oil and thyme provide anti-inflammatory benefits. Garlic adds immune-boosting compounds, making this dish both delicious and nutritious.

Mashed Cauliflower and Sweet Potatoes

This creamy and colorful mash combines sweet potatoes and cauliflower for a nutritious twist on a classic comfort food. It's a perfect side dish for any meal and loaded with vitamins and antioxidants.

Serves: 4 | **Prep Time**: 10 minutes | **Cook Time**: 20 minutes | **Equipment Needed**: Large pot, colander, potato masher or blender | **Nutritional Information**: 140 calories (per serving), 3g protein, 25g carbohydrates, 4g fat

Ingredients:

- 2 medium sweet potatoes (about 400g), peeled and cubed
- 1 small head of cauliflower (about 300g), cut into florets
- 2 tablespoons (30ml) olive oil or unsalted butter
- 1/4 cup (60ml) unsweetened almond milk
- 1/2 teaspoon (1g) salt
- 1/4 teaspoon (1g) black pepper
- 1/4 teaspoon (1g) ground cinnamon (optional, for sweetness)

Instructions:

1. Bring a large pot of water to a boil. Add the sweet potatoes and cauliflower, and cook for 15-20 minutes until tender.
2. Drain the vegetables and return them to the pot.
3. Add the olive oil or butter, almond milk, salt, pepper, and cinnamon (if using). Mash with a potato masher or blend with an immersion blender until smooth and creamy.
4. Taste and adjust seasoning as needed. Serve warm.

Chef's Tip:

- For extra flavor, mix in roasted garlic or a sprinkle of fresh herbs like parsley or chives.
- Store leftovers in an airtight container in the fridge for up to 3 days. Reheat gently on the stovetop or in the microwave.

Thyroid Health Note:

Sweet potatoes are rich in beta-carotene and complex carbohydrates, providing energy and supporting immune function. Cauliflower adds fiber and antioxidants, making this mash a nutrient-dense addition to any meal.

Desserts

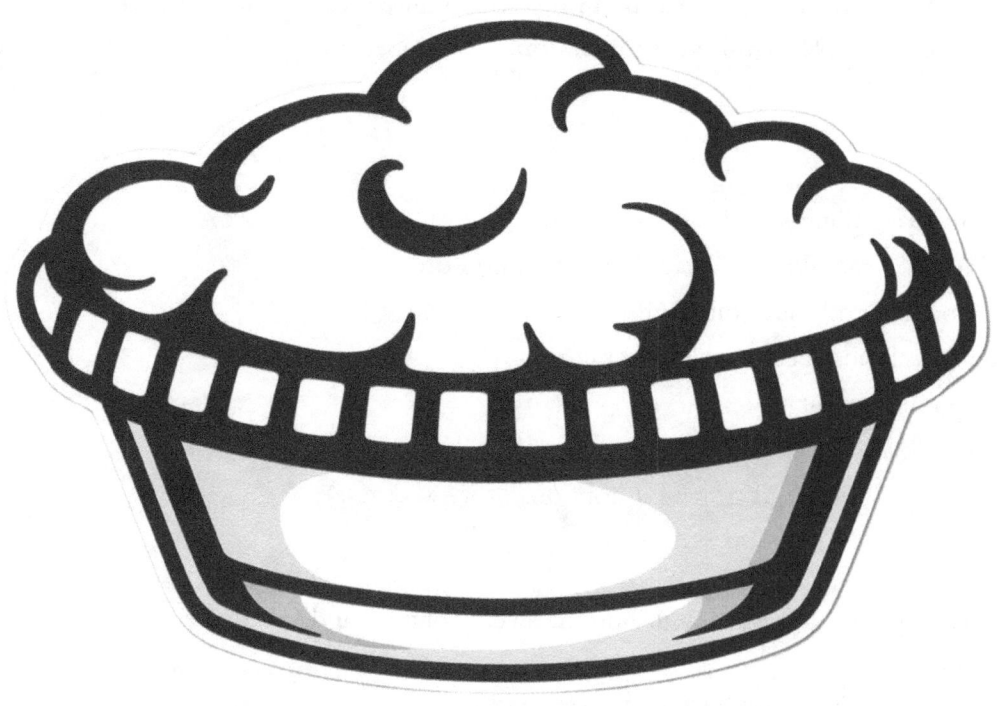

Who says desserts have to be off-limits? With the right ingredients, your sweet indulgences can be both delicious and nourishing. The dessert recipes in this cookbook are crafted to satisfy your cravings while supporting your thyroid health and overall well-being. By choosing natural sweeteners and wholesome ingredients, these treats prove that enjoying a little sweetness doesn't have to come at a cost to your health. Let these recipes inspire you to embrace desserts that are as good for your body as they are for your soul.

Carrot Cake with Almond Flour and Coconut Frosting

This moist and flavorful carrot cake is made with almond flour and topped with a creamy coconut frosting. It's naturally gluten-free and perfect for a special occasion or an everyday treat.

Serves: 8 | **Prep Time**: 15 minutes | **Cook Time**: 35 minutes | **Equipment Needed**: Mixing bowl, whisk, 8-inch round cake pan, grater | **Nutritional Information**: 280 calories (per serving), 6g protein, 20g carbohydrates, 18g fat

Ingredients: For the cake:

- 2 cups (200g) almond flour
- 1 teaspoon (4g) baking soda
- 1/4 teaspoon (1g) ground nutmeg
- 3 large eggs
- 1/4 cup (60ml) melted coconut oil
- 1 cup (100g) grated carrots
- 1/4 cup (30g) coconut flour
- 1/2 teaspoon (2g) ground cinnamon
- 1/4 teaspoon (1g) salt
- 1/3 cup (80ml) maple syrup
- 1 teaspoon (5ml) vanilla extract
- 1/2 cup (50g) chopped walnuts (optional)

For the frosting:

- 1/2 cup (120ml) canned coconut cream (chilled)
- 2 tablespoons (30ml) honey or maple syrup
- 1 teaspoon (5ml) vanilla extract

Instructions

1. Preheat your oven to 350°F (175°C) and grease an 8-inch round cake pan.
2. In a mixing bowl, whisk together the almond flour, coconut flour, baking soda, cinnamon, nutmeg, and salt. In a separate bowl, beat the eggs, maple syrup, melted coconut oil, and vanilla extract until well combined.
3. Gradually add the dry ingredients to the wet ingredients, mixing until a smooth batter forms. Fold in the grated carrots and walnuts (if using).
4. Pour the batter into the prepared cake pan and bake for 30-35 minutes, or until a toothpick inserted into the center comes out clean. Let the cake cool completely.
5. To make the frosting, whip the chilled coconut cream, honey or maple syrup, and vanilla extract until smooth and fluffy. Spread over the cooled cake and serve.

Chef's Tip

- For a decorative touch, sprinkle shredded coconut or chopped nuts on top of the frosting.
- Brush the top of the cake with a light syrup made of honey and water before frosting.

Thyroid Health Note: Almond flour provides vitamin E and healthy fats, while coconut cream and oil offer anti-inflammatory benefits. The carrots add beta-carotene, supporting immune function and overall wellness.

Gluten-Free Brownies with Dark Chocolate and Avocado

These rich and fudgy brownies use avocado for a creamy texture and dark chocolate for a decadent flavor. Naturally gluten-free and low in refined sugars, they're perfect for satisfying your sweet tooth.

Serves: 9 | **Prep Time**: 10 minutes | **Cook Time**: 25 minutes | **Equipment Needed**: Mixing bowl, whisk, 8x8-inch baking pan | **Nutritional Information**: 200 calories (per serving), 4g protein, 15g carbohydrates, 14g fat

Ingredients

- 1 large ripe avocado (about 150g), mashed
- 2 large eggs
- 1/2 cup (100g) coconut sugar
- 1/3 cup (30g) unsweetened cocoa powder
- 1/2 cup (90g) dark chocolate chips (dairy-free if needed), melted
- 1/4 cup (60ml) melted coconut oil
- 1 teaspoon (5ml) vanilla extract
- 1/4 cup (30g) almond flour
- 1/4 teaspoon (1g) salt

Instructions

1. Preheat your oven to 350°F (175°C) and line an 8x8-inch baking pan with parchment paper.
2. In a mixing bowl, mash the avocado until smooth. Add the eggs, coconut sugar, cocoa powder, melted chocolate, coconut oil, and vanilla extract. Mix until well combined.
3. Fold in the almond flour and salt until a smooth batter forms.
4. Pour the batter into the prepared baking pan and spread it evenly. Bake for 20-25 minutes, or until the top is set and a toothpick inserted into the center comes out with a few moist crumbs.
5. Let the brownies cool completely in the pan before slicing into squares.

Chef's Tip

- Add a handful of chopped walnuts or extra chocolate chips to the batter for added texture.
- To intensify the chocolate flavor, add a pinch of espresso powder to the batter.

Thyroid Health Note

Avocado provides healthy fats and magnesium, while dark chocolate is rich in antioxidants that reduce oxidative stress. Coconut sugar offers a lower glycemic alternative to refined sugar, making these brownies both delicious and supportive of thyroid health.

Blueberry Muffins with Coconut Flour

These light and fluffy blueberry muffins are made with coconut flour, making them naturally gluten-free and packed with fiber. They're perfect for a quick breakfast or a healthy snack.

Serves: 6 | **Prep Time:** 10 minutes | **Cook Time:** 20 minutes | **Equipment Needed:** Muffin tin, mixing bowl, whisk | **Nutritional Information:** 160 calories (per muffin), 5g protein, 12g carbohydrates, 10g fat

Ingredients

- 1/4 cup (30g) coconut flour
- 1/4 teaspoon (1g) baking soda
- 1/4 teaspoon (1g) salt
- 3 large eggs
- 1/4 cup (60ml) melted coconut oil
- 3 tablespoons (45ml) maple syrup
- 1 teaspoon (5ml) vanilla extract
- 1/2 cup (75g) fresh or frozen blueberries

Instructions

1. Preheat your oven to 350°F (175°C) and grease or line a muffin tin.
2. In a mixing bowl, whisk together the coconut flour, baking soda, and salt. In a separate bowl, beat the eggs, melted coconut oil, maple syrup, and vanilla extract until smooth.
3. Gradually add the dry ingredients to the wet ingredients, mixing until a thick batter forms. Fold in the blueberries.
4. Divide the batter evenly among 6 muffin cups and bake for 18-20 minutes, or until the tops are golden and a toothpick inserted into the center comes out clean.
5. Let the muffins cool in the tin for 5 minutes before transferring to a wire rack to cool completely.

Chef's Tip

- For a lemony twist, add the zest of 1 lemon to the batter.
- For extra texture, sprinkle a few oats or sliced almonds on top of each muffin before baking.

Thyroid Health Note

Coconut flour is high in fiber and low in carbohydrates, supporting stable blood sugar levels. Blueberries provide antioxidants that reduce inflammation, making these muffins both tasty and thyroid-friendly.

Chia Seed Pudding with Almond Milk and Fresh Fruit

This creamy chia seed pudding is a nutritious and versatile breakfast or snack option. Made with almond milk and topped with fresh fruit, it's naturally gluten-free and packed with fiber and omega-3s.

Serves: 2 | **Prep Time**: 5 minutes | **Chill Time**: 4 hours | **Equipment Needed**: Mixing bowl, whisk, airtight container | **Nutritional Information**: 200 calories (per serving), 5g protein, 15g carbohydrates, 12g fat

Ingredients

- 1/4 cup (40g) chia seeds
- 1 cup (240ml) unsweetened almond milk
- 1 tablespoon (15ml) maple syrup or honey
- 1/2 teaspoon (2.5ml) vanilla extract
- 1/2 cup (75g) fresh fruit (e.g., berries, banana slices, or kiwi)

Instructions

1. In a mixing bowl, whisk together the chia seeds, almond milk, maple syrup, and vanilla extract until well combined.
2. Pour the mixture into an airtight container and refrigerate for at least 4 hours or overnight, stirring once after the first hour to prevent clumping.
3. Before serving, stir the pudding and divide it between two bowls. Top with fresh fruit and enjoy.

Chef's Tip

- Add a sprinkle of cinnamon or a handful of chopped nuts for extra flavor and crunch.
- Make a batch in advance for easy meal prep; the pudding will keep in the fridge for up to 5 days.

Thyroid Health Note

Chia seeds are rich in omega-3s and fiber, supporting heart and thyroid health. Almond milk provides calcium and vitamin E, while fresh fruit adds antioxidants for reducing inflammation.

Banana and Almond Butter Ice Cream

This creamy, dairy-free ice cream is made with just a few simple ingredients and no added sugar. The natural sweetness of bananas pairs perfectly with almond butter for a refreshing and healthy treat.

Serves: 2 | **Prep Time**: 5 minutes | **Freeze Time**: 2 hours | **Equipment Needed**: Food processor or blender | **Nutritional Information**: 180 calories (per serving), 4g protein, 22g carbohydrates, 8g fat

Ingredients

- 2 ripe bananas (about 200g), sliced and frozen
- 2 tablespoons (30g) almond butter
- 1/2 teaspoon (2.5ml) vanilla extract
- A pinch of salt

Instructions

1. Place the frozen banana slices, almond butter, vanilla extract, and salt into a food processor or blender.
2. Blend until smooth and creamy, scraping down the sides as needed.
3. Serve immediately for a soft-serve texture, or transfer to a container and freeze for 1-2 hours for a firmer consistency.
4. Scoop into bowls and enjoy.

Chef's Tip

- For extra flavor, sprinkle with dark chocolate shavings or toasted coconut flakes.
- Freeze individual portions in silicone molds for a convenient grab-and-go snack.

Thyroid Health Note

Bananas are a great source of potassium and energy, while almond butter provides healthy fats and magnesium, both essential for hormone production and thyroid function.

No-Bake Cheesecake with a Date and Nut Crust

This no-bake cheesecake is creamy, rich, and naturally sweetened with dates. The nut-based crust and dairy-free filling make it a guilt-free dessert that's perfect for any occasion.

Serves: 8 | **Prep Time**: 20 minutes | **Chill Time**: 4 hours | **Equipment Needed**: Food processor, 8-inch springform pan | **Nutritional Information**: 280 calories (per serving), 6g protein, 20g carbohydrates, 18g fat

Ingredients

For the crust:

- 1 cup (150g) pitted Medjool dates
- 1 cup (120g) raw almonds or walnuts
- 1/4 teaspoon (1g) salt

For the filling:

- 1 1/2 cups (360g) dairy-free cream cheese
- 1/3 cup (80ml) maple syrup
- 1/4 cup (60ml) coconut cream (chilled)
- 1 teaspoon (5ml) vanilla extract
- Juice of 1/2 lemon (about 1 tablespoon or 15ml)

Instructions

1. In a food processor, blend the dates, almonds, and salt until the mixture sticks together when pressed. Press the mixture evenly into the bottom of an 8-inch springform pan to form the crust.
2. In a mixing bowl, beat the cream cheese, maple syrup, coconut cream, vanilla extract, and lemon juice until smooth and creamy.
3. Pour the filling over the crust and smooth the top with a spatula.
4. Cover the pan and refrigerate for at least 4 hours, or until set.
5. Slice and serve chilled, garnished with fresh fruit or a drizzle of maple syrup if desired.

Chef's Tip

- For a chocolate twist, mix 2 tablespoons of cocoa powder into the filling.
- Store leftovers in the fridge for up to 3 days or freeze individual slices for longer storage.

Thyroid Health Note

The nut-based crust provides healthy fats and selenium, while the coconut cream and dairy-free filling offer anti-inflammatory benefits. This cheesecake is a delightful treat that aligns with thyroid-friendly eating.

Baked Apple with Cinnamon and Chopped Nuts

This simple yet delicious baked apple recipe is warm, comforting, and packed with natural sweetness. Perfect for dessert or a mid-day treat, it's naturally gluten-free and supports thyroid health.

Serves: 2 | **Prep Time**: 5 minutes | **Cook Time**: 25 minutes | **Equipment Needed**: Baking dish, knife, spoon | **Nutritional Information**: 150 calories (per serving), 2g protein, 25g carbohydrates, 6g fat

Ingredients

- 2 medium apples (about 300g), cored
- 2 tablespoons (15g) chopped walnuts or pecans
- 1 teaspoon (2g) ground cinnamon
- 1 tablespoon (15ml) maple syrup or honey
- 1 teaspoon (5g) coconut oil

Instructions

1. Preheat your oven to 375°F (190°C) and grease a small baking dish with coconut oil.
2. Place the cored apples in the baking dish. Fill each apple with chopped nuts and sprinkle with cinnamon.
3. Drizzle maple syrup or honey over the apples and top each with a small dot of coconut oil.
4. Bake for 20-25 minutes, or until the apples are tender and easily pierced with a fork.
5. Serve warm, optionally topped with a dollop of coconut yogurt or a sprinkle of granola.

Chef's Tip

- For added flavor, mix a pinch of nutmeg or ginger with the cinnamon.
- Use different nuts or seeds, like almonds or sunflower seeds, for variation.

Thyroid Health Note

Apples provide fiber and natural sweetness, while walnuts add omega-3s to reduce inflammation. Cinnamon helps regulate blood sugar, making this dish both delicious and nourishing.

Coconut Yogurt with Gluten-Free Granola and Honey

This quick and easy recipe is perfect for breakfast or a light snack. Creamy coconut yogurt paired with crunchy granola and a drizzle of honey makes for a balanced and thyroid-friendly option.

Serves: 2 | **Prep Time**: 5 minutes | **Equipment Needed**: Bowl, spoon | **Nutritional Information**: 180 calories (per serving), 3g protein, 20g carbohydrates, 8g fat

Ingredients

- 1 cup (240g) coconut yogurt
- 1/2 cup (50g) gluten-free granola
- 2 teaspoons (10ml) honey
- 1/4 cup (40g) fresh berries (optional, for topping)

Instructions

1. Divide the coconut yogurt evenly between two bowls.
2. Top each bowl with gluten-free granola and drizzle with honey.
3. Add fresh berries on top, if desired, and serve immediately.

Chef's Tip

- For extra flavor, sprinkle with shredded coconut or a dash of cinnamon.
- Swap honey for maple syrup or agave nectar for a vegan option.

Thyroid Health Note

Coconut yogurt provides healthy fats and probiotics for gut health, while granola adds fiber to support digestion. The honey and berries contribute antioxidants, making this dish both simple and beneficial.

Dark Chocolate and Dried Fruit Bars

These no-bake dark chocolate and dried fruit bars are a rich and satisfying treat, perfect for an afternoon pick-me-up. Packed with antioxidants and healthy fats, they're both indulgent and nourishing.

Serves: 8 | **Prep Time**: 10 minutes | **Chill Time**: 1 hour | **Equipment Needed**: Mixing bowl, 8x8-inch pan, parchment paper | **Nutritional Information**: 220 calories (per serving), 3g protein, 18g carbohydrates, 15g fat

Ingredients

- 1 cup (150g) dark chocolate chips (dairy-free if needed)
- 1/2 cup (50g) chopped mixed dried fruits (e.g., apricots, cranberries, raisins)
- 1/4 cup (25g) chopped almonds or cashews
- 1 tablespoon (15ml) coconut oil
- 1/4 teaspoon (1g) salt

Instructions

1. Line an 8x8-inch pan with parchment paper.
2. Melt the dark chocolate chips and coconut oil in a microwave-safe bowl or over a double boiler, stirring until smooth.
3. Stir in the dried fruits, nuts, and salt until evenly coated with the chocolate.
4. Pour the mixture into the prepared pan, spreading it out evenly. Refrigerate for at least 1 hour, or until firm.
5. Slice into 8 bars and serve chilled or at room temperature.

Chef's Tip

- For extra texture, sprinkle the top with shredded coconut or chia seeds before chilling.
- Store in the fridge for up to 1 week or freeze for longer storage.

Thyroid Health Note

Dark chocolate is rich in antioxidants, while dried fruits provide natural sweetness and vitamins. Nuts add healthy fats and selenium, supporting thyroid function and overall energy.

Beverages

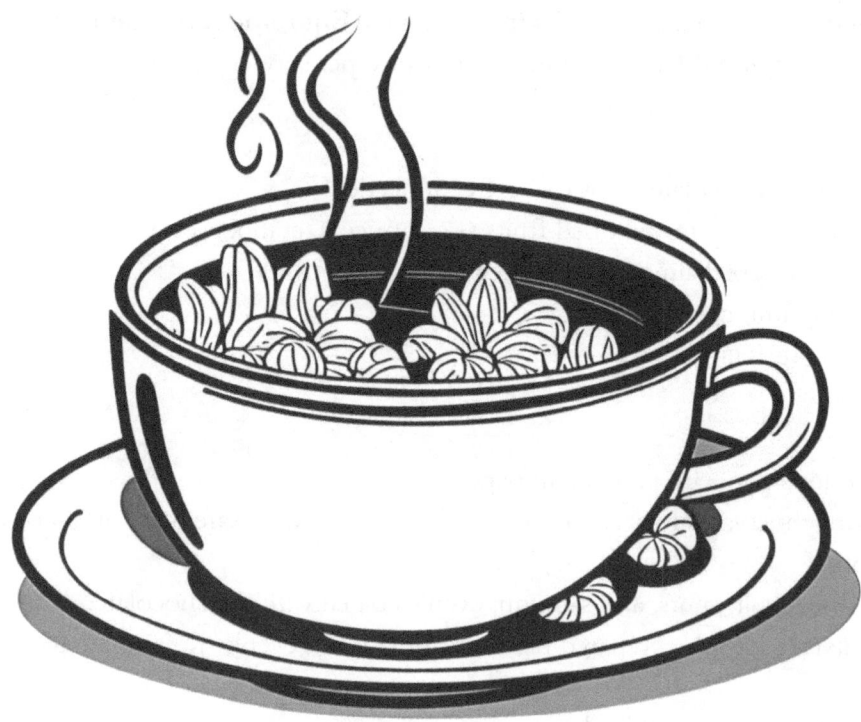

I believe that what you drink is just as important as what you eat, and I'm thrilled to share these beverage recipes with you. From soothing teas to energizing smoothies and refreshing infusions, each drink is designed to nourish your body and support your thyroid health. Whether you're starting your morning or winding down in the evening, these recipes will help you stay hydrated and balanced while enjoying every sip. Let's raise a glass to your well-being!

Ginger and Turmeric Tea with Lemon

This soothing and anti-inflammatory tea combines the power of ginger and turmeric with the refreshing zing of lemon. Perfect for a calming start to your day or a relaxing evening wind-down.

Serves: 2 | **Prep Time**: 5 minutes | **Cook Time**: 10 minutes | **Equipment Needed**: Small pot, knife, grater | **Nutritional Information**: 15 calories (per serving), 0g protein, 4g carbohydrates, 0g fat

Ingredients

- 2 cups (480ml) water
- 1-inch (2.5cm) piece of fresh ginger, grated
- 1/2 teaspoon (1g) ground turmeric or 1-inch (2.5cm) fresh turmeric, grated
- Juice of 1/2 lemon (about 1 tablespoon or 15ml)
- 1 teaspoon (5ml) honey (optional)

Instructions

1. Bring the water to a boil in a small pot.
2. Add the grated ginger and turmeric, reduce heat, and simmer for 10 minutes.
3. Strain the tea into two cups and stir in the lemon juice. Add honey if desired.
4. Serve immediately and enjoy warm.

Chef's Tip

- For added flavor, sprinkle a pinch of black pepper into the tea to enhance turmeric's absorption.

Thyroid Health Note

Ginger and turmeric are potent anti-inflammatory ingredients, while lemon provides vitamin C for immune support. This tea is an excellent way to boost circulation and promote overall wellness.

Mint and Cucumber Infusion

This refreshing infusion combines cool cucumber and invigorating mint for a hydrating beverage that's perfect for hot days or as a light detox drink.

Serves: 4 | **Prep Time**: 5 minutes | **Chill Time**: 1 hour | **Equipment Needed**: Large pitcher, knife | **Nutritional Information**: 5 calories (per serving), 0g protein, 1g carbohydrates, 0g fat

Ingredients

- 1 medium cucumber (about 200g), thinly sliced
- 1/4 cup (10g) fresh mint leaves
- 1 liter (4 cups) water
- Juice of 1/2 lime (about 1 tablespoon or 15ml)

Instructions

1. Add the cucumber slices and mint leaves to a large pitcher.
2. Pour in the water and lime juice, stirring gently to combine.
3. Refrigerate for at least 1 hour to allow the flavors to infuse.
4. Serve chilled, garnished with additional mint leaves if desired.

Chef's Tip

- Add a few slices of lemon or a handful of crushed berries for a fruity twist.
- Keep the infusion refrigerated and consume within 2 days for optimal freshness.

Thyroid Health Note

Cucumber is hydrating and helps flush toxins, while mint supports digestion and provides a refreshing flavor. This drink is a simple yet effective way to stay hydrated and energized.

Anti-Inflammatory Smoothie with Pineapple and Turmeric

This vibrant smoothie is loaded with anti-inflammatory ingredients like pineapple and turmeric, making it a delicious and nourishing choice for any time of day.

Serves: 1 | **Prep Time**: 5 minutes | **Equipment Needed**: Blender | **Nutritional Information**: 200 calories (per serving), 3g protein, 35g carbohydrates, 6g fat

Ingredients

- 1 cup (165g) fresh or frozen pineapple chunks
- 1/2 teaspoon (1g) ground turmeric
- 1/2 cup (120ml) unsweetened almond milk
- 1/2 cup (120ml) water
- 1/2 teaspoon (1g) grated fresh ginger
- Juice of 1/2 orange (about 2 tablespoons or 30ml)
- A handful of ice cubes (optional)

Instructions

1. Add all the ingredients to a blender and blend until smooth.
2. Taste and adjust sweetness if needed by adding a small amount of honey or maple syrup.
3. Serve immediately, garnished with a sprinkle of turmeric or a wedge of orange.

Chef's Tip

- For added creaminess, replace half of the almond milk with coconut milk.

Thyroid Health Note

Pineapple provides bromelain, an enzyme with anti-inflammatory properties, while turmeric and ginger support immune function and reduce oxidative stress. This smoothie is a powerful, thyroid-friendly drink.

Protein Smoothie with Spinach, Almond Butter, and Flaxseeds

This creamy, protein-packed smoothie is a perfect meal replacement or post-workout option. With spinach, almond butter, and flaxseeds, it delivers sustained energy and essential nutrients.

Serves: 1 | **Prep Time**: 5 minutes | **Equipment Needed**: Blender | **Nutritional Information**: 300 calories (per serving), 15g protein, 20g carbohydrates, 18g fat

Ingredients

- 1 cup (30g) fresh spinach leaves
- 1 tablespoon (16g) almond butter
- 1 tablespoon (10g) ground flaxseeds
- 1/2 frozen banana (about 50g)
- 1 scoop (30g) vanilla plant-based protein powder
- 1 cup (240ml) unsweetened almond milk
- A handful of ice cubes (optional)

Instructions

1. Add all the ingredients to a blender and blend until smooth and creamy.
2. Adjust the consistency by adding more almond milk if needed.
3. Serve immediately and enjoy cold.

Chef's Tip

- Add a pinch of cinnamon or nutmeg for extra flavor.

Thyroid Health Note

Spinach provides magnesium and iron, while almond butter and flaxseeds offer healthy fats and omega-3s. Combined with protein powder, this smoothie supports muscle repair and thyroid function.

Part 4: Lifestyle Strategies for Thriving

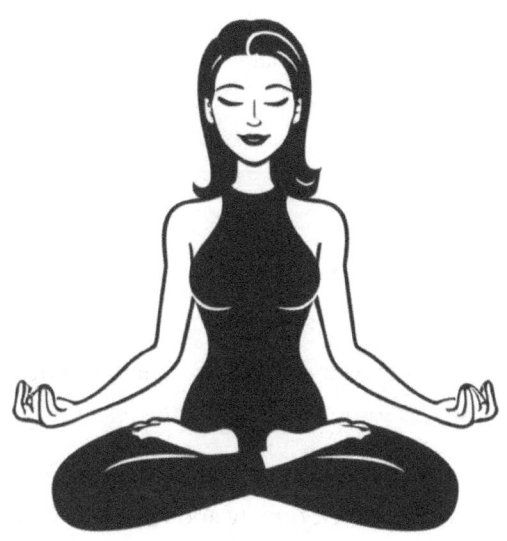

Stress and Hashimoto's

How Stress Affects Your Thyroid

Stress is an inevitable part of life, but when it becomes chronic, it can wreak havoc on your thyroid and overall health. For individuals with Hashimoto's, chronic stress amplifies inflammation, disrupts hormonal balance, and worsens symptoms, making stress management a cornerstone of healing. Chronic stress doesn't just affect the mind—it triggers a chain reaction throughout your body that directly impacts thyroid function.

When you're under stress, your body releases cortisol, a hormone produced by the adrenal glands. While cortisol is essential in small doses for managing immediate challenges, chronic stress keeps cortisol levels elevated, overwhelming your endocrine system. This disruption can suppress thyroid hormone production, inhibit the conversion of T4 (inactive hormone) to T3 (active hormone), and increase systemic inflammation, intensifying autoimmune activity.

As cortisol levels remain elevated, symptoms such as fatigue, brain fog, difficulty concentrating, and weight gain become more pronounced. Research shows that chronic stress also weakens the immune system's ability to regulate itself, prolonging inflammation and making it harder to manage Hashimoto's effectively. For example, stress can create a vicious cycle—heightened inflammation worsens symptoms, which in turn increases stress, further disrupting thyroid function.

Example: Lisa, one of my closest childhood friends, a mother balancing a demanding job and family responsibilities, noticed her Hashimoto's symptoms spiraling out of control during a particularly stressful work project. Her fatigue deepened, and her ability to concentrate diminished. When she started incorporating short mindfulness exercises and daily walks in nature, she began to feel more energized and less overwhelmed, breaking the stress cycle.

Stress also impacts sleep, digestion, and emotional resilience, making it essential to implement stress management strategies tailored to your needs.

Techniques for Stress Reduction

Managing stress doesn't require overhauling your entire life. Small, intentional actions can significantly reduce stress and support thyroid health. Here are some effective strategies:

Mindfulness and Meditation: Even five to ten minutes a day can make a difference. Apps like Headspace or Calm offer guided meditations, but you can also sit quietly and focus on your breath. Deep breathing calms your nervous system, lowers cortisol, and enhances mental clarity. For instance, taking five slow, deep breaths before starting a stressful task can help you approach it with a calmer mindset. Incorporate body scan meditations or progressive muscle relaxation to further release tension. These practices guide you in focusing on each part of your body, promoting both physical and mental relaxation.

Relaxing Physical Activities: Gentle exercises such as yoga, tai chi, or leisurely walks in a park combine movement with relaxation. Studies show that yoga reduces cortisol levels, improves flexibility, and enhances overall well-being. Walking in nature, often called "forest bathing," has also been shown to lower stress hormones and increase feelings of calm. Experiment with restorative yoga, which focuses on deep stretching and relaxation, or tai chi movements that emphasize slow, mindful motions to cultivate balance and inner peace.

Journaling: Writing down your thoughts and emotions helps identify stress triggers and provides emotional release. Try keeping a gratitude journal by writing three positive things about your day each evening. This practice shifts focus from stress to appreciation, reducing anxiety over time. Use journaling prompts to explore deeper emotional patterns, such as "What situations tend to trigger stress for me?" or "What small victories did I achieve today?" Journaling can also help clarify goals and foster a sense of control.

Breathing Techniques: Diaphragmatic breathing is a powerful, simple tool for immediate stress relief. Inhale through your nose for a count of four, hold for four, and exhale through your mouth for six. Repeating this for a few minutes can bring an immediate sense of calm, even in high-pressure moments. Explore techniques like alternate nostril breathing (nadi shodhana), which balances the nervous system, or box breathing (inhale-hold-exhale-hold for equal counts) for enhanced focus and relaxation.

Prioritize Self-Care: Engaging in hobbies you love—whether reading, gardening, or crafting—provides a mental reset. Scheduling these moments of joy is not indulgent but an essential act of self-preservation. Dedicate specific "self-care slots" in your weekly calendar and treat them as non-negotiable appointments with yourself. Use this time to recharge and reconnect with what brings you happiness.

Social Connection: Building a strong support network can buffer the effects of stress. Share your challenges with trusted friends, family, or support groups who understand your journey with Hashimoto's. Meaningful connections foster resilience and reduce feelings of isolation. Join local or online communities dedicated to thyroid health, where you can exchange tips, share experiences, and find encouragement from others navigating similar challenges.

Limit Exposure to Stress Triggers: Identify stressors within your control, such as an overpacked schedule or constant notifications on your phone. Set boundaries and establish clear limits to protect your mental well-being. Implement a "digital detox" by turning off notifications during meals or designated relaxation periods. Creating a technology-free zone in your home can also foster a more calming environment.

By integrating these techniques into your daily life, you can build a sustainable framework for managing stress and improving your thyroid health. From my own experience and countless conversations with others navigating Hashimoto's, I've learned that consistency is key—small daily efforts truly compound over time to create significant improvements. Stress is an inevitable part of life, but how you choose to respond to it can make all the difference in your healing journey. I'm certain that the strategies shared here will empower you to take control and find a sense of calm. And for those looking to dive deeper, the bonus section at the end of this book provides additional resources and insights on advanced stress management strategies tailored to support your unique path to wellness.

Sleep and Recovery

The Role of Rest in Healing

Sleep is the foundation of health, particularly for those with Hashimoto's. It's during sleep that your body repairs tissues, regulates hormones, and fortifies the immune system—all critical for managing autoimmune conditions. Unfortunately, many individuals with Hashimoto's struggle with sleep disturbances, further exacerbating their symptoms.

Sleep deprivation disrupts hormonal balance, leading to increased cortisol levels, reduced energy production, and heightened systemic inflammation. These physiological changes amplify symptoms such as fatigue, brain fog, and difficulty maintaining a healthy weight. Research highlights that those sleeping fewer than six hours a night experience significantly worse Hashimoto's symptoms compared to individuals who consistently get seven to nine hours of sleep.

Poor sleep also impacts emotional well-being, increasing susceptibility to anxiety and depression. Over time, this creates a cycle where poor sleep worsens symptoms, and worsening symptoms make restful sleep harder to achieve. It's a frustrating loop that many people feel powerless to break, but it's important to remember that even small changes can make a big difference. Prioritizing high-quality sleep is one of the most impactful steps you can take to support your thyroid health and overall vitality.

Why Sleep is Critical for Hashimoto's

When you sleep, your body engages in numerous processes that directly support thyroid health and immune system function. During deep sleep, the body reduces cortisol levels, which helps decrease systemic inflammation—a key driver of Hashimoto's symptoms. Additionally, sleep promotes the release of growth hormone, essential for tissue repair and cellular regeneration, both of which are critical for thyroid healing.

Sleep also supports brain health, improving cognitive function and memory consolidation. This is particularly important for individuals with Hashimoto's, who often experience brain fog and difficulty concentrating. Without adequate rest, the brain's ability to process information and regulate emotions becomes impaired, increasing susceptibility to anxiety and depression. A well-rested mind is better equipped to handle the challenges of managing a chronic condition like Hashimoto's.

Tips for Better Sleep Hygiene

Improving sleep doesn't require drastic changes. Small adjustments to your routine and sleep environment can make a profound difference. Here are some strategies to help you create an environment and routine conducive to restful sleep:

Establish a Pre-Sleep Routine: A calming ritual before bed helps signal to your body that it's time to unwind. This could include light stretching, journaling, or listening to soothing music. Avoid screens for at least an hour before bed, as the blue light emitted by devices disrupts melatonin production, the hormone responsible for regulating sleep. For example, Mark, a teacher managing Hashimoto's, replaced evening screen time with reading a physical book and noticed a significant improvement in his sleep quality. Adding mindfulness practices, such as deep breathing exercises or a short meditation, can further relax your mind and body, setting the stage for restorative sleep.

Optimize Your Sleep Environment: Transform your bedroom into a true sanctuary for sleep. Blackout curtains can block out intrusive light, while maintaining a cool room temperature between 60-67°F promotes deeper sleep cycles. A supportive mattress and pillows tailored to your comfort preferences can reduce physical tension, helping you fall asleep faster and stay asleep longer. Enhancing the atmosphere with soothing elements like lavender essential oils, white noise machines, or soft, breathable bedding can create a cocoon of relaxation.

Consider Natural Supplements: Certain supplements may help improve sleep quality, but it's essential to consult a healthcare provider before introducing anything new. Magnesium, often called "nature's relaxant," can ease muscle tension and promote calmness. Melatonin can assist with falling asleep but should be used sparingly to avoid dependence. Herbal teas, such as chamomile or valerian root, can be part of a comforting nightly ritual, gently signaling to your body that it's time to rest.

Stick to a Schedule: Consistency is one of the most effective ways to improve sleep. Going to bed and waking up at the same time every day—even on weekends—reinforces your body's internal clock, making it easier to fall asleep and wake up feeling refreshed. Sarah, a busy professional, found success by setting a "wind-down alarm" at 9:30 p.m., which reminded her to dim the lights, sip chamomile tea, and journal. Over time, this routine became second nature, and her sleep quality improved dramatically.

Limit Stimulants: Caffeine, alcohol, and heavy meals in the evening can interfere with your body's ability to wind down. Instead, opt for light snacks like a banana or a handful of nuts, which provide nutrients like magnesium and tryptophan to support relaxation and sleep. Drinking a warm, caffeine-free herbal tea can also help signal to your body that bedtime is approaching.

Incorporate Movement During the Day: Gentle physical activity during the day can promote better sleep at night. Activities like walking, yoga, or tai chi reduce stress and prepare your body for rest. However, avoid vigorous exercise close to bedtime, as it can elevate cortisol levels and make it harder to relax.

Creating a Sustainable Sleep Framework

Improving sleep is not just about what happens at night; it's about setting the stage throughout your day. From establishing calming routines to optimizing your sleep environment, these strategies build the foundation for high-quality rest. Remember, sleep and stress management go hand in hand: better sleep reduces stress, and managing stress promotes more restful sleep.

I know from personal experience and from working with others that improving sleep takes time and persistence, but the rewards are well worth it. Restful sleep provides the energy, mental clarity, and emotional resilience needed to tackle the challenges of managing Hashimoto's. For additional tips and advanced strategies, refer to the bonus section at the end of this book, where I've included tools and resources to help you further refine your approach to sleep and recovery. Together, these small but powerful changes can help you reclaim your health and restore your vitality.

Exercise for Energy

The Right Workouts for Hashimoto's

Exercise is a powerful tool for supporting overall health and managing Hashimoto's, but not all workouts are created equal. For individuals with Hashimoto's, choosing the right types of exercise is essential to avoid overexertion and support energy levels. When done thoughtfully, exercise can help regulate hormones, reduce inflammation, and improve overall vitality.

Low-impact exercises like walking, yoga, and stretching are ideal for those with limited energy. These activities promote circulation, reduce stress, and enhance flexibility without placing undue strain on the body. For example, Sarah, a working professional with Hashimoto's, found that a gentle 20-minute evening walk not only improved her mood but also reduced her fatigue over time. Research supports these observations, showing that yoga can reduce cortisol levels by up to 25% while improving overall flexibility and reducing inflammation. Incorporating even a short daily walk can boost cardiovascular health, enhance mood, and lower systemic inflammation, making it an accessible and effective option for most individuals.

In addition to low-impact activities, incorporating light resistance training into your routine is also crucial. Resistance exercises, such as bodyweight movements or using light dumbbells, help maintain muscle mass, support bone density, and improve metabolism. Research indicates that even 15 minutes of light resistance training twice a week can significantly boost muscle strength and metabolic health without causing overexertion. Simple movements like squats, lunges, or push-ups performed two to three times a week can help build strength and resilience, ensuring your body stays supported as you manage Hashimoto's.

Even on days when energy levels are particularly low, short sessions of movement can make a meaningful difference. Stretching for five minutes or performing a few restorative yoga poses can enhance mobility, relieve tension, and promote relaxation. The key is to listen to your body and adapt your routine to align with your current energy levels. Movement doesn't have to be strenuous to be beneficial; every small step contributes to overall health and recovery.

Listening to Your Body: How to Avoid Overexertion

Exercise is beneficial, but overdoing it can backfire, particularly for those managing Hashimoto's. Recognizing the signs of overexertion and balancing activity with recovery is vital for maintaining long-term health and preventing unnecessary setbacks.

Persistent muscle soreness, excessive fatigue after workouts, and difficulty recovering between sessions are common indicators that you may be pushing too hard. For instance, Mark, an enthusiastic runner, noticed that his intense training sessions left him drained for days, making it harder to maintain his routine. By switching to shorter, low-intensity sessions, he was able to rebuild his energy levels while maintaining his fitness. This underscores the importance of pacing yourself and adapting your routine to meet your body's current needs.

Balancing exercise and recovery requires a gradual and patient approach. Start with short, low-intensity sessions and increase duration or intensity as your stamina improves. For example, begin with 10-minute walks and gradually extend them to 20 or 30 minutes over several weeks. Progressing slowly ensures that your body can adapt without becoming overwhelmed, reducing the risk of burnout.

Incorporating rest days into your schedule is equally important. These days give your body time to heal and replenish energy stores, which is particularly crucial for managing Hashimoto's. Rest days don't mean complete inactivity—activities like restorative yoga, gentle stretching, or even slow-paced walks can keep you active while promoting recovery. By allowing your body the time it needs to recover, you build a sustainable routine that supports long-term health.

Creating an Exercise Routine That Works for You

Developing an exercise routine tailored to your needs and energy levels is key to maximizing the benefits of movement while managing Hashimoto's. Here are some practical strategies to create a balanced routine:

1. **Set Realistic Goals:** Begin with small, achievable objectives, such as walking for 10 minutes a day or incorporating one yoga session per week. Celebrate these milestones to build confidence and motivation.
2. **Mix It Up:** Variety in your exercise routine keeps it engaging and helps target different aspects of health. Combine low-impact cardio with light resistance training and stretching for a well-rounded approach.
3. **Track Your Progress:** Keeping a journal or using an app to log your workouts can help you monitor your energy levels and identify patterns. This information is invaluable for adjusting your routine to better suit your needs.
4. **Prioritize Recovery:** Listen to your body and don't hesitate to take additional rest days if needed. Recovery is just as important as the exercise itself in building strength and resilience.
5. **Seek Support:** Join a class, hire a trainer familiar with autoimmune conditions, or connect with a supportive community to stay motivated and accountable.

Exercise, when approached thoughtfully, is a powerful ally in managing Hashimoto's. It helps regulate hormones, reduce inflammation, and improve overall energy levels. By choosing activities that align with your body's needs and incorporating rest and recovery, you can create a sustainable exercise routine that supports both your physical and emotional well-being. Remember, progress is not about perfection—it's about consistently showing up for yourself in ways that feel good and promote healing. For additional tips and resources on creating a personalized exercise plan, refer to the bonus section at the end of this book, where you'll find tools and strategies to further refine your approach.

Detox Your Environment

Reducing Exposure to Toxins

Environmental toxins can interfere with thyroid function and exacerbate autoimmune activity. Reducing your exposure to these harmful substances is an important step in managing Hashimoto's and supporting overall health. While it's impossible to completely eliminate toxins from your environment, small, intentional changes can make a significant impact over time.

Common toxins that affect thyroid health include pesticides, heavy metals like mercury and lead, and chemicals found in plastics, such as BPA. According to the Environmental Working Group (EWG), BPA exposure has been linked to disruptions in endocrine function, including thyroid hormone regulation. To reduce exposure, start by making practical changes in your daily life. For example, switching from plastic food containers to glass or stainless steel can prevent harmful chemicals from leaching into your meals. Choosing organic produce whenever possible can also help minimize pesticide intake. If buying all organic isn't feasible, focus on the EWG's "Dirty Dozen" list of the most pesticide-laden fruits and vegetables.

Synthetic fragrances and harsh cleaning products are another common source of toxins. Many air fresheners, candles, and household cleaners contain endocrine-disrupting chemicals that can interfere with thyroid health. Replacing these products with natural alternatives can create a safer home environment. For instance, using an essential oil diffuser instead of chemical-laden air fresheners helped Emily, a mother with Hashimoto's, significantly reduce her family's exposure to harmful substances while maintaining a pleasant and inviting home. Similarly, switching to unscented, natural detergents and household cleaners, such as those made with vinegar and baking soda, can drastically lower your toxic load. These simple, cost-effective solutions are both safer and environmentally friendly.

Filtering your water is another simple yet effective step to reduce exposure to harmful substances. Unfiltered water can contain chlorine, heavy metals, and other impurities that may contribute to thyroid dysfunction over time. According to a report by the CDC, regular exposure to these contaminants can strain the thyroid and overall endocrine system. Installing a high-quality water filter, whether for your faucet or a whole-house system, can remove chlorine, lead, and other pollutants, providing cleaner water for drinking, cooking, and bathing. This simple change not only supports thyroid health but also promotes better overall wellness.

Choosing Clean Products

Switching to clean, non-toxic products is one of the most effective ways to reduce your exposure to harmful substances and protect your thyroid. Begin by evaluating the products you use in your home and personal care routine. For household cleaning, natural alternatives like castile soap, vinegar, and baking soda are not only effective but also safe for your family and the environment. For example, Lisa, who was concerned about the chemical exposure her children faced, started using castile soap for cleaning surfaces and found peace of mind knowing she was creating a healthier home environment.

When it comes to personal care, look for cosmetics and skincare products free from parabens, phthalates, sulfates, and synthetic fragrances. Many clean beauty brands now prioritize transparency, making it easier to identify safe options. Switching to a natural deodorant or a shampoo without sulfates is a small change that can reduce your exposure to potentially harmful chemicals over time. Look for certifications like "EWG Verified" or "USDA Organic" to ensure you're choosing products with clean ingredients.

Filtering your water should also be a priority. Beyond drinking water, consider how the water you bathe and cook with impacts your body. Installing a whole-house filtration system or even a simple shower filter can reduce your exposure to chlorine, heavy metals, and other impurities, providing a cleaner environment for your skin and hair while supporting internal health.

Simple Steps to Detoxify Your Environment

Detoxifying your environment doesn't require drastic changes. Instead, focus on small, consistent efforts that compound over time. Here are some actionable steps you can take:

1. **Reduce Plastic Use:** Opt for glass or stainless steel containers for food and water storage. Avoid microwaving food in plastic containers to prevent chemical leaching.
2. **Choose Organic When Possible:** Prioritize organic options for produce, dairy, and meat to minimize pesticide and hormone exposure. Use the EWG's "Clean Fifteen" and "Dirty Dozen" lists as guides for budgeting organic purchases.
3. **Switch to Natural Cleaners:** Replace conventional cleaning products with natural alternatives like vinegar, baking soda, and castile soap. Essential oil-based sprays can also freshen up your space without introducing synthetic chemicals.
4. **Eliminate Synthetic Fragrances:** Ditch air fresheners, candles, and perfumes with synthetic fragrances. Use essential oils in a diffuser for a healthier and equally pleasant alternative.
5. **Filter Your Water:** Invest in a high-quality water filtration system for drinking and cooking, and consider a shower filter to reduce exposure to chlorine and other chemicals.
6. **Be Mindful of Personal Care:** Choose shampoos, deodorants, and skincare products that are free from harmful additives like parabens, phthalates, and sulfates. Start by replacing one item at a time to make the transition manageable.

Detoxifying your environment is a journey, not a one-time event. By making intentional choices about the products you use and the substances you allow into your home, you can significantly reduce your toxic load and support your thyroid health. I've seen firsthand how these changes, though small at first, can lead to profound improvements over time. Remember, it's not about perfection but progress. For those eager to explore this topic further, the bonus section at the end of this book provides detailed resources and tools to help you create a cleaner, healthier living environment. These efforts, combined with other lifestyle strategies, will empower you to reclaim your health and thrive.

Part 5: Resources and Tools

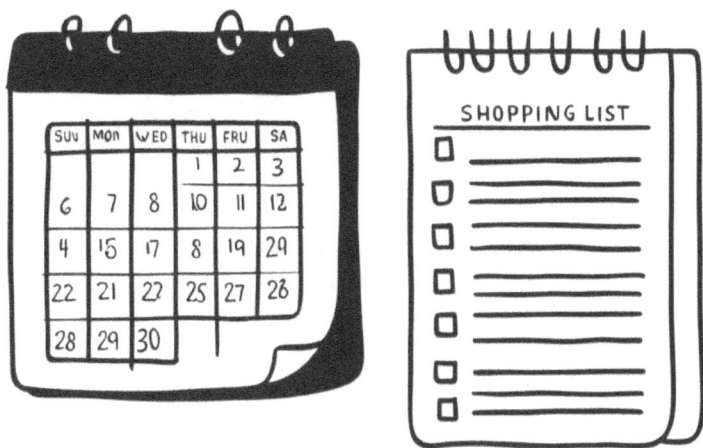

28 Weekly Meal Plans | Shopping Lists

Congratulations on taking the first step toward reclaiming your health and embracing a lifestyle that supports your well-being! This chapter is designed to provide you with a carefully crafted 28-day meal plan, tailored to simplify your journey toward balanced eating and managing Hashimoto's. Whether you're new to meal planning or seeking a structured guide, this plan will serve as the perfect starting point.

Why This Meal Plan?

The 28-day meal plan included here is a tool to help you kickstart your dietary transformation with ease. It was created with careful attention to balance macronutrients, offer variety, and include the delicious recipes from this book. Each meal has been chosen to nourish your body, support your thyroid health, and reduce inflammation—all while keeping your taste buds satisfied.

Empowering You to Create Your Own Plan

While this meal plan provides a ready-to-use solution, my ultimate goal is to empower you. The educational content throughout this book will equip you with the tools and knowledge to craft your own meal plans, tailored to your preferences, dietary needs, and lifestyle. You'll learn how to balance meals, select thyroid-supportive ingredients, and adjust your plan to suit your unique journey.

Access Printable Meal Plans and Shopping Lists

To make your experience even more convenient, you'll find bonus materials included with this book. By scanning the QR code or visiting the link provided, you'll have access to a printable version of the 28-day meal plan and **shopping lists**, perfect for placing on your fridge or taking with you on grocery trips. Additionally, there are exclusive content and resources to further support your journey, which you'll discover through the QR code or link.

You're On Your Way!

By following this plan, you're not just adopting a new way of eating—you're embracing a lifestyle that prioritizes your health and vitality. Be proud of the effort you've made to care for yourself. As you move forward, remember that every small choice adds up to a big impact on your well-being.

Now, let's dive into your meal plan and start this journey together. Here's to a healthy, thriving you!

1 Weekly Meal Plan

	BREAKFAST	LUNCH	DINNER
MON	GREEN SMOOTHIE WITH KALE, AVOCADO, AND FLAXSEEDS	QUINOA BOWL WITH GRILLED SALMON	SWEET POTATO AND LENTIL SHEPHERD'S PIE
TUE	TROPICAL SMOOTHIE WITH PINEAPPLE, GINGER, AND COCONUT MILK	RED LENTIL CURRY SOUP WITH COCONUT MILK	HERB-ROASTED CHICKEN WITH SWEET POTATOES
WED	PROTEIN SMOOTHIE WITH ALMOND BUTTER AND BLUEBERRIES	SEASONAL VEGETABLE MINESTRONE WITH BONE BROTH	MOROCCAN CHICKPEA TAGINE WITH APRICOTS AND ALMONDS
THU	ALMOND FLOUR PANCAKES WITH NATURAL MAPLE SYRUP	ROASTED CHICKEN SALAD WITH AVOCADO AND SUNFLOWER SEEDS	ZUCCHINI LASAGNA WITH TURKEY AND SPINACH
FRI	COCONUT FLOUR WAFFLES WITH FRESH BERRIES	VEGETARIAN BUDDHA BOWL WITH SPICED CHICKPEAS AND HUMMUS	GARLIC BUTTER SHRIMP WITH ZUCCHINI NOODLES
SAT	OATMEAL BOWL WITH CHIA SEEDS AND CINNAMON	SLOW-COOKED BEEF POT ROAST WITH ROOT VEGETABLES	SLOW-COOKED BEEF POT ROAST WITH ROOT VEGETABLES
SUN	SPINACH, AVOCADO, AND SUN-DRIED TOMATO FRITTATA	BAKED CHICKEN AND VEGETABLE STEW	INDIAN-SPICED LENTIL DHAL WITH COCONUT RICE

2 Weekly Meal Plan

	BREAKFAST	LUNCH	DINNER
MON	SCRAMBLED EGGS WITH MUSHROOMS AND CARAMELIZED ONIONS	SHRIMP SCAMPI WITH SPAGHETTI SQUASH	EGGPLANT AND CHICKPEA STEW WITH TOMATOES AND SPICES
TUE	SWEET POTATO TOAST WITH HUMMUS AND AVOCADO	QUINOA BOWL WITH GRILLED SALMON	THAI GREEN CURRY WITH VEGETABLES AND COCONUT MILK
WED	GREEN SMOOTHIE WITH KALE, AVOCADO, AND FLAXSEEDS	LENTIL AND SWEET POTATO PATTIES	LEMON-BAKED SALMON WITH BROCCOLI AND CAULIFLOWER
THU	TROPICAL SMOOTHIE WITH PINEAPPLE, GINGER, AND COCONUT MILK	ROASTED CHICKEN SALAD WITH AVOCADO AND SUNFLOWER SEEDS	MUSHROOM AND SPINACH RISOTTO (DAIRY-FREE)
FRI	PROTEIN SMOOTHIE WITH ALMOND BUTTER AND BLUEBERRIES	GARLIC BUTTER SHRIMP WITH ZUCCHINI NOODLES	MOROCCAN CHICKPEA TAGINE WITH APRICOTS AND ALMONDS
SAT	ALMOND FLOUR PANCAKES WITH NATURAL MAPLE SYRUP	SEASONAL VEGETABLE MINESTRONE WITH BONE BROTH	HERB-ROASTED CHICKEN WITH SWEET POTATOES
SUN	COCONUT FLOUR WAFFLES WITH FRESH BERRIES	BAKED CHICKEN AND VEGETABLE STEW	SPANISH-STYLE GARLIC SHRIMP (GAMBAS AL AJILLO)

3 Weekly Meal Plan

	BREAKFAST	LUNCH	DINNER
MON	OATMEAL BOWL WITH CHIA SEEDS AND CINNAMON	RED LENTIL CURRY SOUP WITH COCONUT MILK	SWEET POTATO AND LENTIL SHEPHERD'S PIE
TUE	SPINACH, AVOCADO, AND SUN-DRIED TOMATO FRITTATA	QUINOA BOWL WITH GRILLED SALMON	SHRIMP SCAMPI WITH SPAGHETTI SQUASH
WED	SCRAMBLED EGGS WITH MUSHROOMS AND CARAMELIZED ONIONS	VEGETARIAN BUDDHA BOWL WITH SPICED CHICKPEAS AND HUMMUS	THAI GREEN CURRY WITH VEGETABLES AND COCONUT MILK
THU	SWEET POTATO TOAST WITH HUMMUS AND AVOCADO	LENTIL AND SWEET POTATO PATTIES	ZUCCHINI LASAGNA WITH TURKEY AND SPINACH
FRI	GREEN SMOOTHIE WITH KALE, AVOCADO, AND FLAXSEEDS	GARLIC BUTTER SHRIMP WITH ZUCCHINI NOODLES	MUSHROOM AND SPINACH RISOTTO (DAIRY-FREE)
SAT	ALMOND FLOUR PANCAKES WITH NATURAL MAPLE SYRUP	SLOW-COOKED BEEF POT ROAST WITH ROOT VEGETABLES	MOROCCAN CHICKPEA TAGINE WITH APRICOTS AND ALMONDS
SUN	PROTEIN SMOOTHIE WITH ALMOND BUTTER AND BLUEBERRIES	EGGPLANT AND CHICKPEA STEW WITH TOMATOES AND SPICES	HERB-ROASTED CHICKEN WITH SWEET POTATOES

4 Weekly Meal Plan

	BREAKFAST	LUNCH	DINNER
MON	ALMOND FLOUR PANCAKES WITH NATURAL MAPLE SYRUP	BAKED CHICKEN AND VEGETABLE STEW	CAULIFLOWER STEAK WITH CHIMICHURRI SAUCE
TUE	COCONUT FLOUR WAFFLES WITH FRESH BERRIES	QUINOA BOWL WITH GRILLED SALMON	LEMON-BAKED SALMON WITH BROCCOLI AND CAULIFLOWER
WED	OATMEAL BOWL WITH CHIA SEEDS AND CINNAMON	ROASTED CHICKEN SALAD WITH AVOCADO AND SUNFLOWER SEEDS	INDIAN-SPICED LENTIL DHAL WITH COCONUT RICE
THU	SPINACH, AVOCADO, AND SUN-DRIED TOMATO FRITTATA	SHRIMP SCAMPI WITH SPAGHETTI SQUASH	ZUCCHINI LASAGNA WITH TURKEY AND SPINACH
FRI	SCRAMBLED EGGS WITH MUSHROOMS AND CARAMELIZED ONIONS	VEGETARIAN BUDDHA BOWL WITH SPICED CHICKPEAS AND HUMMUS	THAI GREEN CURRY WITH VEGETABLES AND COCONUT MILK
SAT	SWEET POTATO TOAST WITH HUMMUS AND AVOCADO	GARLIC BUTTER SHRIMP WITH ZUCCHINI NOODLES	SWEET POTATO AND LENTIL SHEPHERD'S PIE
SUN	GREEN SMOOTHIE WITH KALE, AVOCADO, AND FLAXSEEDS	SEASONAL VEGETABLE MINESTRONE WITH BONE BROTH	SPANISH-STYLE GARLIC SHRIMP (GAMBAS AL AJILLO)

Conversion Chart: US Customary, Imperial, and Metric Systems

Weight

US Customary	Imperial	Metric
1 ounce (oz)	1 ounce (oz)	28 grams (g)
8 ounces (1/2 pound)	8 ounces	227 grams (g)
16 ounces (1 pound)	16 ounces (1 pound)	454 grams (g)
2 pounds	2 pounds	907 grams (g)

Volume (Liquid)

US Customary	Imperial	Metric
1 teaspoon (tsp)	1 teaspoon (tsp)	5 milliliters (ml)
1 tablespoon (tbsp)	1 tablespoon (tbsp)	15 milliliters (ml)
1 fluid ounce (fl oz)	1 fluid ounce (fl oz)	30 milliliters (ml)
1 cup	8 fluid ounces	240 milliliters (ml)
1 pint	20 fluid ounces	473 milliliters (ml)
1 quart	40 fluid ounces	946 milliliters (ml)
1 gallon	160 fluid ounces	3.8 liters (L)

Volume (Dry)

US Customary	Imperial	Metric
1/4 cup	N/A	60 milliliters (ml)
1/3 cup	N/A	80 milliliters (ml)
1/2 cup	N/A	120 milliliters (ml)
2 cups (1 pint)	N/A	480 milliliters (ml)
4 cups (1 quart)	N/A	950 milliliters (ml)

Temperature

US Customary	Imperial	Metric
32°F	32°F	0°C
212°F	212°F	100°C
N/A	N/A	Formula: (°F - 32) × 5/9 = °C

Conclusion

As we reach the end of this book, I want to take a heartfelt moment to thank you for allowing me to walk alongside you on this journey. Writing this book has been a deeply personal labor of love, inspired by my belief that no one should have to face the challenges of Hashimoto's alone. I hope these pages have been more than just a guide—I hope they've felt like a companion, offering you support, encouragement, and a path forward.

This is not the end—it's the start of a beautiful new chapter in your life. Healing and thriving with Hashimoto's may not always be easy, but every small step you take—whether it's preparing a nourishing meal, embracing a moment of self-care, or simply acknowledging your progress—is a victory worth celebrating. You are stronger and more resilient than you may realize, and you deserve to live a life of energy, balance, and joy.

As you move forward, I encourage you to explore the additional resources and bonuses I've prepared for you. They're designed to support you further on this path, with practical tools and thoughtful inspiration to make your journey even smoother.

Thank you for trusting me to be part of your story. Know that I am cheering for you every step of the way. My greatest wish is for you to feel empowered, vibrant, and deeply connected to the life you are building. Here's to your health, your happiness, and the incredible journey ahead.

Bonus

I'm so happy to offer you a little extra support on your journey to better health!

Just scan the QR code with your phone's camera to find bonus meal plans, extra recipes, and simple tools to make your path to wellness even easier and more enjoyable.

With love,

Mary Walker

Made in United States
Cleveland, OH
11 November 2025

25830236R00066